Color Atlas of Urology

Second Edition

R W Lloyd-Davies
MS, FRCS, FEBU
Senior Consultant Surgeon
Department of Urology
St Thomas's Hospital
London
Clinical Director of Urology and Lithotripsy
Guy's and St Thomas's Hospital Trust
Past President of the Section of Urology of the Royal Society of Medicine

H Parkhouse
FRCS, FRCS(Urol), FEBU
Consultant Urologist
Mount Vernon and Hillingdon Hospitals
London

J G Gow
MD, ChM, FRCS
Consultant Urologist (Emeritus)
Liverpool Area Health Authority Teaching
Past President of the Section of Urology of the Royal Society of Medicine

D R Davies
MB, BS, MRCS, LRCP, FRCPath
Consultant Pathologist
John Radcliffe Hospital
Oxford
Formerly Reader in Histopathology, UMDS, and Consultant Pathologist, St Thomas's Hospital

NWolfe

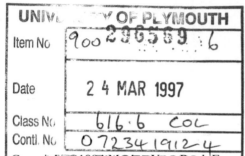
Copyright © 1994 Mosby–Year Book Europe Limited
Published in 1994 by Wolfe Publishing, an imprint of Mosby–Year Book Europe Limited
Printed by Grafos, S. A. Arte sobre papel
ISBN 0 7234 19124

For full details of all Mosby–Year Book Europe Limited titles, please write to Mosby–Year Book Europe Limited, Lynton House, 7–12 Tavistock Square, London WC1H 9LB, England.

A CIP catalogue record for this book is available from the British Library.

Library of Congress Cataloging-in-Publication Data has been applied for.

Contents

Preface to the second edition

The original concept of the Atlas was twofold: first to reacquaint urologists and general surgeons with common and uncommon urological conditions and secondly to emphasise that urology is a broad subject embracing many other medical disciplines, which are essential for efficient patient management and which are complementary to good urological practice.

Ten years have elapsed since the first edition was published and during that time the advances in investigative procedures and urological techniques have been striking and imaginative and have improved the prospects of recovery and rehabilitation for patients. Nevertheless, the second edition has endeavoured to preserve the original objectives.

Although the original format has been retained, there have been many changes. There is one new author, Mrs Helen Parkhouse, a Consultant Urologist with a special interest in Paediatric Urology, and she is warmly welcomed. The chapter on congenital deformities has been completely rewritten. Magnetic resonance imaging (MRI) and positron emission tomography (PET) have been included among the investigative procedures, and ureterorenoscopy has been incorporated because of its importance in the diagnosis and treatment of upper urinary tract pathology. Corpora cavernosography is another investigation that has given new dimensions to the management of impotence. The pathogenesis of urinary stone disease has been revised and there is a short comment on human immunodeficiency virus (HIV) and urology because it is a subject which is very pertinent to present-day urological practice. We appreciate that there may still be omissions but we hope that this new edition will assist with the problems of clinical reasoning, which can only be of outstanding and abiding advantage to every patient.

Preface to the first edition

Urology, arguably the oldest speciality, has now assumed its rightful place in the forefront of surgical practice, as it embraces 30 per cent of all surgical problems. As in the last two decades significant progress has been made in all branches of urology, it can no longer be considered within the precincts of the general surgeon, although until further expansion of urological appointments has taken place, it is accepted that many urological cases will have to be treated by general surgeons throughout the world.

This book is therefore aimed at a comprehensive readership embracing senior clinical students, junior urologists at all stages of their training and general surgeons with an interest in urology. It is hoped also that the practising urologist will find something of value, because we have attempted to include many of the results of the exciting scientific advances which have taken place in urology in recent years.

Much of the information is basic; for this we make no apology, because we consider it is fundamental to have a sound knowledge of first principles.

Successful diagnosis is based on a combination of clinical acumen and the interpretation of appropriate investigations. We have combined investigations, macropathology and histopathology with normal and special stains and where appropriate endoscopic photography to emphasise the importance of interdisciplinary co-operation in urology.

The first chapter is therefore a description of standard urological investigations, together with tables of normal values which can be used as a reference to compare results obtained in various pathological conditions.

In recent years urodynamics has begun to play an ever-increasing role in the investigation of disorders of micturition; consequently this diagnostic procedure has been included in some detail.

The discovery by Professor Hopkins of the rod lens system and the flexible glass fibre bundles has revolutionised endoscopy. It is now possible to portray with sufficient detail and accurate colour rendering, lesions in the urethra and bladder. A considerable part of this book has been devoted to this aspect of urology, so that endoscopists can become more readily acquainted with the normal and abnormal appearances of the urethra and bladder.

The boundary between urology and nephrology is often obscure and deceptive and we are conscious that we may have trespassed into the territory of the nephrologists. However, we feel that if a true understanding is to be achieved it is impossible not to invade the ground more properly assigned to them, and if in doing so we have made unacceptable errors, we ask for their understanding.

In this book we have attempted to include as many as possible of the commoner conditions and some of the rare diseases. It is not meant, however, to compete with textbooks of urology but to complement them and to be appreciated as a pictorial record encompassing a broad spectrum of urology.

We have not sought in any way to cover paediatric urology and have made only brief mention of renal failure and venereology and trauma, because we considered they were not subjects suitable to this kind of presentation.

Because it is an atlas the introductory texts and legends are short and are used only to highlight the more important points of each illustration.

We hope that the atlas will be treated not just as a reference but will act as a stimulus to provoke the reader to delve deeper into the many exciting projects which have now become part of the practice of urology.

In such a book there will be many omissions particularly among the rarer diseases; for this we can only crave the indulgence of the reader and hope that it may be possible to correct them in subsequent editions.

Acknowledgements to the second edition

We have carried out a very thorough revision to create the second edition of this Atlas, which incorporates not only the modalities of investigation that have undergone considerable development in the past 10 years, but also those that are new techniques. We are therefore very grateful to our colleagues who have given help and advice, and would like particularly to thank Dr B.A. Ayers and Dr D. Rickards, who reviewed all the ultrasound and CT scans throughout the book. Dr Rickards also provided the new Doppler studies. Dr T. Nunan reviewed all the radioisotope material and added the PET studies, Dr C.I. Meanock advised over MRI and contributed the MRI scans, Dr C.S. Bradbeer contributed the section on HIV and urology, and Mr R.S. Cole revised and expanded the chapter on Urinary Tract Stones. Mr W.T. Lawrence provided the comparative slides of flexible and rigid cystoscopy, and Professor M.A. Ghoneim of Mansoura, Egypt reviewed the chapter on Schistosomiasis and contributed some further slides. To these colleagues, whose contributions have led to a completely new look to this book, we are deeply indebted.

We wish to thank the many colleagues listed below for the loan of the new illustrations used in this edition.

Dr B.A. Ayers **1, 2, 5, 6, 12–16, 18, 27, 35, 36, 42–44, 330, 331, 720–722, 787–790, 794–796, 854–857, 1057, 1058, 1243–1245, 1249, 1255, 1256, 1276.**

Dr T.D. Bates **1287, 1288.**

Dr C.S. Bradbeer **395–397.**

Mr R.S. Cole **561, 562, 567–574, 579, 580, 582–585, 592, 595–598, 605, 606, 616, 617, 634, 635, 640, 643, 645, 646, 650–654, 656, 659, 686, 693, 694.**

Professor M.A. Ghonheim **501, 502, 511, 515.**

Mr N.W. Harrison **244.**

Mr W.T. Lawrence **96, 97, 105, 106, 877, 878, 882, 1015, 1016.**

Dr L.M. MacDonald **138–142, 172, 173, 218, 219.**

Dr C.I. Meanock **45–47, 722–726, 730, 731, 749–751, 777, 778, 791, 891, 908, 1273, 1274.**

Dr T.O. Nunan **60–67, 203, 205, 276, 277, 279, 554, 825, 848, 849, 1068, 1289, 1290.**

Mr E.P. O'Donoghue **1050.**

Mr P.G. Ransley **240, 245–247, 249.**

Dr D. Rickards **8–11, 50, 58, 59, 656, 927, 928, 975, 1051–1053, 1171–1174, 1176, 1177, 1263–1266.**

Mr K.A. Woolfenden **51–54, 627–629.**

Miss Amanda German of the Central Illustration Services of UMDS St Thomas's Hospital has been responsible for the revision and creation of the artwork throughout the new edition.

This new edition could not have been completed without the very considerable secretarial help of Mrs Julie Roe. She has been fully involved in the revision of this edition, and to her go our very sincere thanks.

Acknowledgements to the first edition

We are very grateful to our colleagues, without whose help and encouragement this Atlas could not have been completed. Mr K.E.D. Shuttleworth, Mr N.O.K. Gibbon, Mr R.M. Jamieson and Mr M.R. Heal have contributed a large range of Diagnostic problems, and Mr M.I. Bultitude has been particularly helpful with the section on Urodynamics. Dr A. Carty, Dr N.H. Crosby, Dr J.H.E Carmichael, Dr A.B. Ayers, Dr M. Lea-Thomas and Dr J. Pemberton, our Radiological colleagues, have been very helpful, and to them we are most appreciative.

Dr A.B. Ayers in addition has given a notable contribution to the ultrasound studies. Dr E.W. Lupton has been most generous in supplying the Renograms, and we are very indebted to him. We also thank Mr W.B. Peeling and his colleagues Mr P.J. Brooman, Dr G.H. Griffiths, Dr K.T. Evans and Mr E.E. Roberts for their help with the new technique of transrectal ultrasonography. Bruel and Kjær (UK) Ltd., have generously donated slides **925**, **926** and **929**, illustrating the latest technique for transrectal ultrasonography. Mr F.T. Graves has been very kind in allowing us to use photographs **70, 72–74, 158** and **164**, which are reproduced by permission of John Wright & Son, Bristol, and F.T. Graves, in whose monograph, *The Arterial Anatomy of the Kidney, the basis of Surgical Technique,* further details of the intrarenal vascular system can be found.

We wish to thank the many colleagues listed below for the loan of illustrations. Dr M. Black and his colleagues of The Department of Dermatology, St Thomas's Hospital (**1221, 1222**); Mr N. Blackford; Mr M.I. Bultitude (**122–135**); Dr R.D. Catterall (**1087**); Mr P.B. Clark (**365, 964**); Dr C.D. Collins (**1282, 1283**); Professor El Ghorab and Dr N. Badr for providing most of the non-histological Bilharzia slides; Mr R. Ewing (**1138**); Dr S. Eykyn (**88,89**); Mr C. Gingell (**1104, 1145, 1167, 1181–1192, 1197, 1202, 1203, 1212, 1214, 1250, 1251, 1254, 1270, 1271**); Mr W.F. Hendry (**1260, 1262**); Dr Eadie Heyderman for the histology sections from which **1305** and **1319** were taken; Mr J.P. Hopewell (**1150**); Professor M.S.R. Hutt (**514**), and for allowing us access to his collection of tropical pathological slides; Mr C.H. Parkinson for the sections from which **871** and **872** were taken; Mr W.B. Peeling and his colleagues (**109, 947**); Dr J. Pincott (**186**); Mr J.M. Pullan (**1286**); The Royal Tropical Institute (**487–492**); Professor J.B. Stewart (**1316**); Mr T.A. Taylor (**1145**); Dr K. Thomas (**1324**); Professor J.R. Tighe (**383**) and for allowing us access to the files of the Histopathology Department, St Thomas's Hospital; and Mr R.H. Whitaker (**68, 69** and **206–209**).

Our thanks are due to Miss Beryl Evans for the preparation of most of the histology slides; Mr V. Clarke for the photography of many of the pathological specimens; Mr T. Brandon and his staff, Photographic Department, St Thomas's Hospital; Mr W.C. Fitzsimmons and his staff, Photographic Department, Liverpool Eastern District and Mr J. Stammers and his staff, Central Photographic Department, University of Liverpool. Mr Ken Biggs, Medical Artist, Anatomy Department, University of Liverpool has been responsible for the line drawings and the excellent colour diagrams, and his superb technique has added considerable distinction to the Atlas.

No work such as this could be completed without the help and sympathetic understanding of our secretaries, Mrs J.E. Stephens, Mrs N.M. Williams, Mrs B.D. Worthington and Miss M. Murphy, and to them we shall always be most grateful.

1 Investigations

One of the primary concerns of any urologist is the investigation and management of patients presenting with haematuria. All such patients will require urine analysis, imaging of their urinary tract, and an endoscopic assessment. Urine examination will include microscopy, culture, and determination of the sensitivity pattern of any organisms; cytology and phase contrast microscopy are also frequently performed.

In terms of imaging the intravenous urogram was the gold standard until the advent of ultrasonography. In recent years the great advances in ultrasound imaging have replaced the more invasive methods of radiology, but there is still a place for both techniques. Ultrasonography is considerably more operator-dependent than radiology, but is noninvasive, carries no hazard, and is of relatively low cost. In very expert hands, particularly when combined with plain abdominal films, it is an extremely valuable screening tool. There is still a body of opinion however that favours radiology, particularly in the investigation of haematuria, despite the fact that it is invasive, expensive, and has side-effects. Death has been

rarely reported as a result of anaphylactic shock. The intravenous urogram probably still has the edge on ultrasonography for providing fine detail of the pelvicalyceal system and ureter, but experts of the latter contest this and it will be interesting to follow further developments over the next 10 years.

Endoscopic assessment of the urethra and bladder is still mandatory in the investigation of haematuria, but inspection with the rigid cystoscope is being increasingly replaced by the use of the flexible instrument.

Ultrasound and flexible cystoscopy now play key parts in the investigation of the urological patient and this has occurred in the 10 years since the publication of the first edition of this book.

In the management of any urological patient there are three main facets.

- First and most important is the history.
- Second is the clinical examination.
- Third is the use of ancillary investigations that are considered appropriate to the clinical assessment.

Renal ultrasound

In the 10 years since the publication of the first edition of this book there have been considerable changes and advances in the investigation and the sequence of investigation of the urological patient. Ultrasound carries the great advantage of being a noninvasive technique based on sonography. It does not require the injection of contrast media when it is used to evaluate cystic and solid renal masses or to localise needles accurately for aspiration, biopsy, or percutaneous nephrostomy. It does not, however, provide any information about renal function.

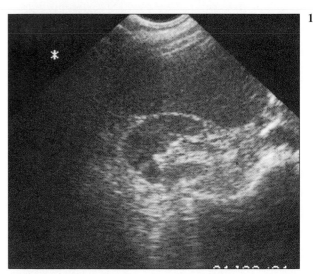

1 Normal transverse ultrasound of renal area.

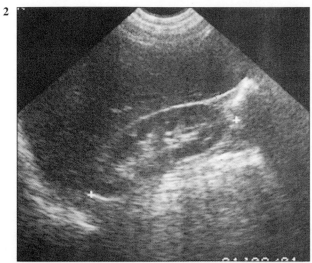

2 Normal longitudinal ultrasound of renal area. A smooth renal outline can be seen together with a slim, pelvicalyceal system.

3 Full male bladder. Note the smooth outline and lack of any evidence of trabeculation, and the prostatic impression in the base.

4 Male bladder study after voiding. There is no significant residual urine.

5 Full female bladder.

6 Female bladder study after voiding.

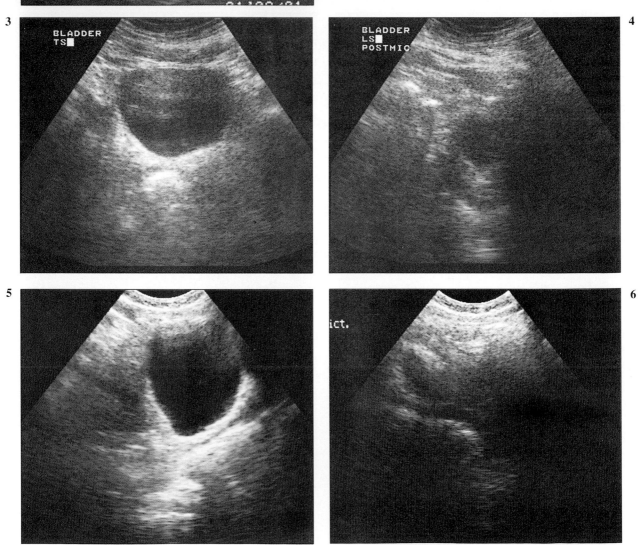

Prostatic imaging by transrectal ultrasonography

The assessment and diagnosis of prostatic disease by rectal palpation can be inaccurate, especially for the smaller nodule. In addition, only the back and posterior lateral parts of the gland are accessible to palpation and to digitally guided needle biopsy.

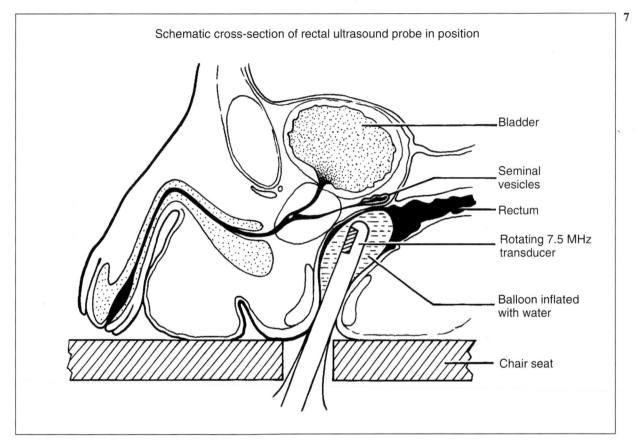

Schematic cross-section of rectal ultrasound probe in position

- Bladder
- Seminal vesicles
- Rectum
- Rotating 7.5 MHz transducer
- Balloon inflated with water
- Chair seat

7 Imaging of the prostate can provide a full ultrasound map of the whole prostate gland and demonstrates the prostatic capsule at all levels. The seminal vesicles and bladder base can be differentiated from the surrounding tissues, allowing measurement of prostatic dimensions. The prostate is imaged with an ultrasound probe with a rotating transducer and introduced through the anal canal so that it enters the lower rectum.

A water-filled balloon surrounds the probe tip and the linear array 7MHz transducer gives a 135° scan of the prostate in all directions. Ultrasonograms of the prostate from the bladder base and seminal vesicles to the prostatic apex can be obtained by withdrawing the probe at 0.5 cm intervals, and ultrasound-guided needle biopsies can be taken from any abnormal or suspicious area.

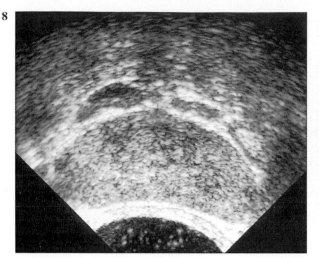

8 Transverse axial transrectal ultrasound of the prostate. The prostate is well defined and predominantly homogeneous. This is an ultrasound of a young man in whom the peripheral zone of the gland accounts for more than 75% of the total gland substance.

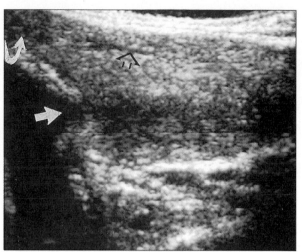

9 Sagittal transrectal ultrasound scan of the prostate. The bladder neck (arrow), seminal vesicle (curved arrow), and ejaculatory duct (open arrow) can be seen.

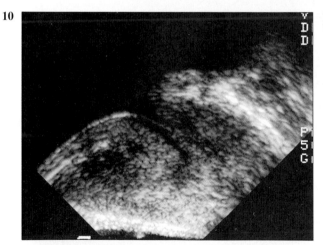

10 Sagittal transrectal ultrasound using the forward looking transducer. The bladder neck and proximal posterior urethra can be seen. This probe is used to guide transrectal biopsy.

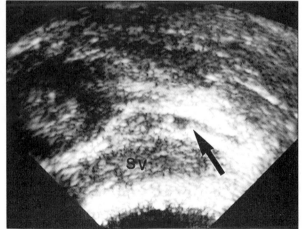

11 Transverse axial transrectal ultrasound at the level of the seminal vesicle. The left vas deferens can be seen entering the seminal vesicle (arrow). SV = seminal vesicle.

Testicular ultrasound

Ultrasonography is a standard investigation in testicular disorders and can accurately demonstrate pathology in the body of the testis distinct from the epididymis. Combined with colour Doppler it will demonstrate vascular abnormalities including torsion and varicocoele.

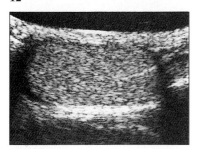

12 Longitudinal scan of testis.

13 Transverse scan of both testes showing an entirely normal echo pattern.

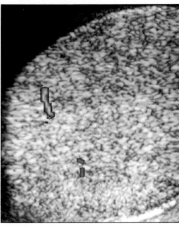

14 Colour Doppler scan of normal testis showing a small amount of blood flow, which is within normal limits.

Radiology

Intravenous urogram (IVU)

The excretory urogram demonstrates anatomical features of the renal parenchyma and pelvicalyceal system and at the same time gives some information about the functional capacity of the whole system. There are two phases. First the nephrogram outlines the upper nephron as much of the water reabsorption occurs in the proximal tubules. This phase demonstrates functional renal tissue and the density of the nephrogram will therefore assist estimation of the quality of glomerular filtration.

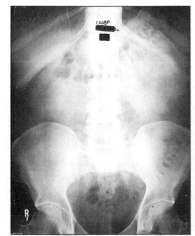

15 A full length plain film taken in inspiration demonstrates the renal outlines and any abnormal opacities in the urinary tract and particularly renal calcification.

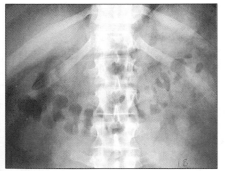

16 A renal film taken in expiration will often demonstrate the outline more satisfactorily because the kidneys are moved away from the costal margin.

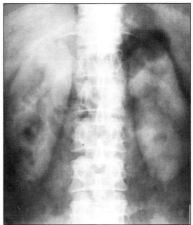

17 Nephrogram showing the outlines of the kidneys.

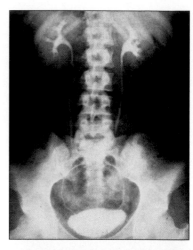

18 Pyelogram. Excretory phase at 10 minutes to show the calyces, pelvis, and upper ureters.

19 Normal IVU. Full length film.

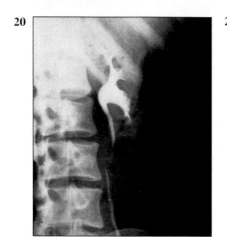

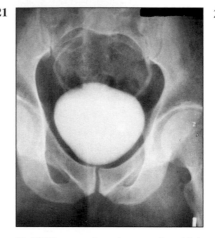

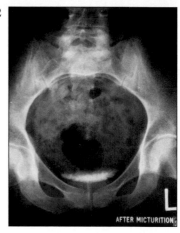

20 An oblique view of a normal upper urinary tract often helps to outline a small calyceal lesion.

21 IVU normal cystogram in which the bladder outline is smooth and regular.

22 IVU normal post-micturition film in which the contrast medium is seen between the folds of the flaccid mucous membrane.

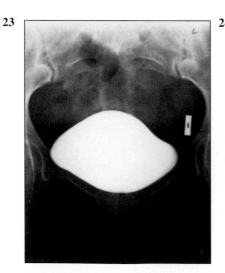

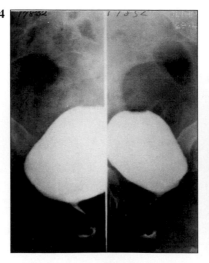

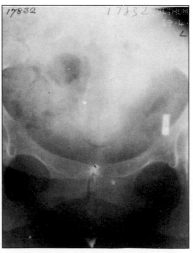

23 Normal micturating cystogram. Female: full bladder.

24 Normal micturating cystogram. Female: during micturition (oblique views to show any reflux).

25 Normal micturating cystogram. Female: after micturition.

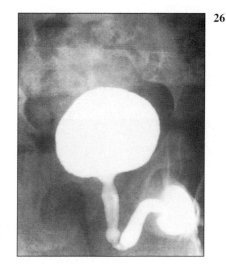

26

26 Normal micturating cystogram.
Male: normal micturating cystogram in a
boy. Note the contrast inside the prepuce.

Tomograms are useful adjuncts to the conventional
urogram in helping to differentiate whether a lesion is in
the anterior, middle, or posterior portion of the kidney,
especially in the presence of intestinal gas.

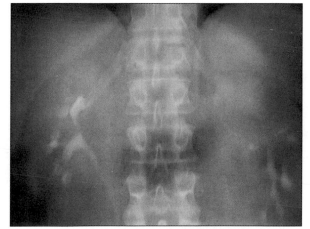

27

27 Tomogram of both kidneys taken at 15 minutes after contrast with a 9 cm cut.

Pyelovenous backflow

What was originally thought to be pyelovenous backflow
is now (with modern high-dose techniques) considered to
be a concentration of contrast medium in the collecting
tubules giving a dense pyramidal outline.

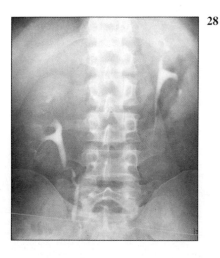

28

28 Dense pyramidal contrast.

Ureterography/retrograde pyelography

This procedure is used less often because of the improved intravenous urographic techniques. When retrograde studies are required they should first be performed through a bulb-ended catheter to allow a dynamic study of the ureter, using the image intensifier at the time of the injection. Later a fine catheter can be passed to the kidney if required.

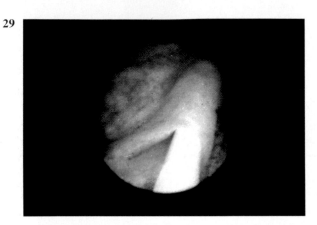

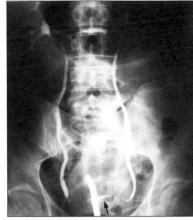

29 Ureterography. Catheter bulb in place in ureteric orifice.

30 Bilateral normal ascending ureterogram. Note the bulb-ended catheter.

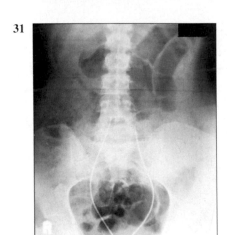

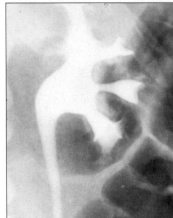

31 Retrograde pyelography. Bilateral retrograde catheters *in situ*.

32 Retrograde pyelography. Fine detail of the pelvicalyceal system.

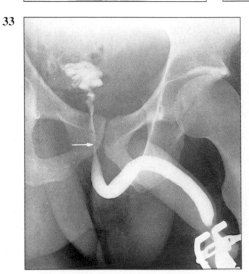

33 Urethrography. Normal ascending urethrogram. The urethra is smooth and always becomes narrow in the region of the external sphincter. The verumontanum is shown as a filling defect in the prostatic urethra.

Arteriography

Selective renal arteriography is carried out by passing a catheter up the femoral artery and guiding it into the renal artery under image intensification. If this method is not possible, the axillary artery or a translumbar aortic puncture may be used.

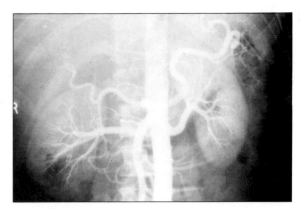

34

34 Flush arteriogram showing the vascular tree and the architecture of both kidneys. It will identify plaques in the renal artery.

Subtraction arteriography

A subtraction arteriogram is useful in assessing the vascular flush of malignant renal tumours because it highlights the vessels in much greater detail.

35 Digital subtracted angiography (DSA). Selective injection into the renal artery on the right.

36 Use of digital subtraction to show the intrarenal arteries clearly.

35 **36**

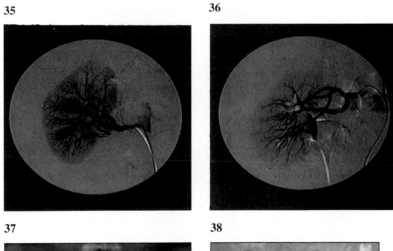

37 Arteriogram of the internal iliac artery showing the pudendal artery. This is an essential investigation in some cases of impotence.

38 Subtraction arteriogram of the internal iliac artery showing the pudendal artery.

37 **38**

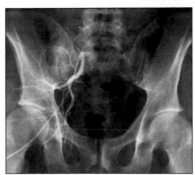 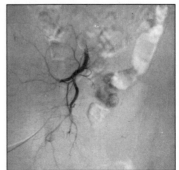

Inferior venocavogram

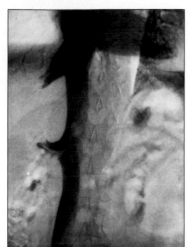

A cavogram may be important for assessing the spread of lesions such as a renal carcinoma because it will show renal vein obstruction or the presence of tumour within the lumen.

39 Normal subtraction cavogram.

Lymphography

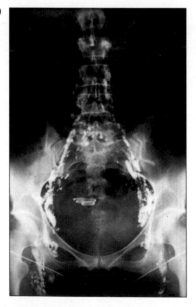

Abdominal lymphography can be used as a guide in the staging of various malignant conditions, such as testicular tumours and carcinoma of the prostate. It is indicated in investigating patients with lymph node enlargement of obscure cause, chyluria, lymphoma, retroperitoneal fibrosis, testicular tumours, carcinoma of the prostate, and carcinoma of the penis. It has been largely replaced by CT scanning.

40 Normal lymphogram.

Seminal vesiculogram

A seminal vesiculogram is occasionally carried out to exclude obstructive lesions in the ejaculatory system, especially those close to the verumontanum.

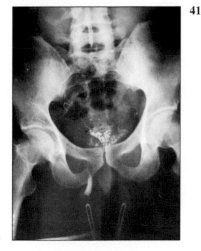

41

41 Normal vesiculogram.

Computerised axial tomography (CT)

CT is reconstruction by computer of a radiographic tomographic image through a particular plane of the body. It is used with intravenous contrast medium to study renal pathology.

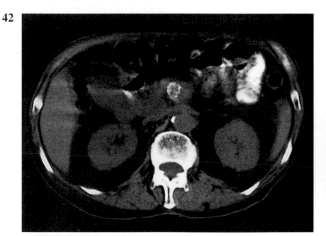
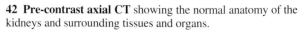

42

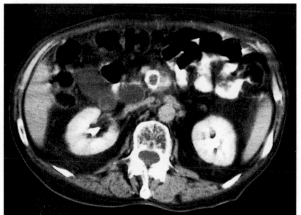

43

42 Pre-contrast axial CT showing the normal anatomy of the kidneys and surrounding tissues and organs.

43 Post-contrast axial CT showing the normal anatomy of the kidneys and surrounding tissues and organs.

44 Post-contrast axial CT demonstrating the renal pelvis and showing the normal anatomy of the kidneys and surrounding tissues and organs.

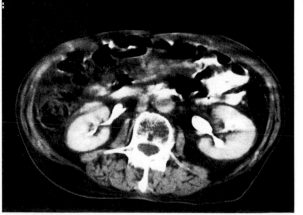

44

Magnetic resonance imaging

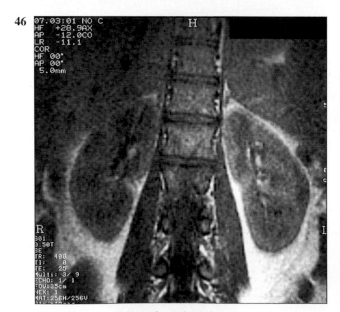

45 MRI study of both kidneys. The axial view shows differentiation between the cortex and medulla.

The application of nuclear magnetic resonance (NMR) to urology is a major innovation. Now widely termed magnetic resonance imaging (MRI) it involves no ionising radiation and its imaging principles differ from those of existing techniques. The MR signal provides not only morphological, but also biochemical detail using spectroscopy.

The information obtained with MRI used in tandem with CT as the modality of choice shows that the two techniques are complementary and each has advantages in different tissues.

The inability of MRI to demonstrate calcification is a major shortcoming with regard to the urinary tract. Its great advantage is the multiplanar imaging of neoplasms, which allows accurate staging.

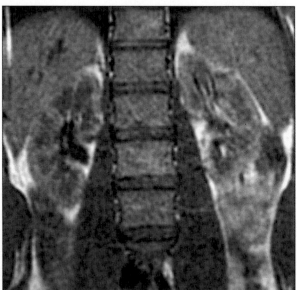

46 MRI coronal view of renal outlines.

47 MRI coronal view showing vessels in renal hilum.

Positron emission tomography

Positron emission tomography (PET) is an advanced imaging technique that allows high resolution images. All the isotopes used have a short half-life, so an on-site cyclotron is necessary. One of the most useful agents is 18-fluorodeoxyglucose (18-FDG). This is a glucose analogue and is used to image tumour sites when other imaging modalities are not helpful. PET imaging shows no isotope uptake in normal tissues. See also Chapter 7, p.184 and Chapter 12, p.280.

Cyst puncture

Cyst puncture is now a normal method of investigating not only the outline of cysts, but also for making a detailed examination of cyst contents and can be performed with either ultrasound or CT.

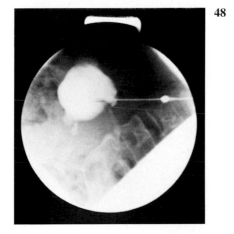

48

48 Normal cyst puncture. This technique is useful in the diagnosis of cystic renal lesions, but has been largely superseded by CT screening.

Renal biopsy

A renal biopsy may be the only way to make an exact diagnosis, but it is not without its hazards.

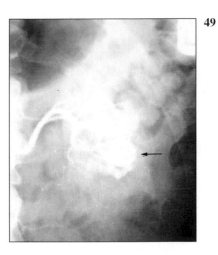

49

49 Arteriovenous fistula after renal biopsy.

Nephrostogram

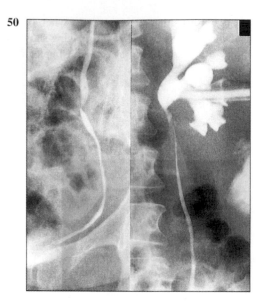

50

50 Percutaneous intubation of the pelvicalyceal system allows imaging with contrast medium of not only the system, but also the whole ureter, and allows drainage of the upper tract.

Ureterorenoscopy

Ureterorenoscopy has become an important diagnostic and therapeutic procedure for many conditions of the upper urinary tract. One important indication for which it can be carried out is ureterolithotomy, either using only endoscopic instruments or in conjunction with lithotripsy. Another indication is the removal of stents that have migrated from the bladder into the ureter.

Both rigid and flexible ureteroscopes are now available and a video camera is a useful addition to the flexible instrument.

Both types of ureteroscopes need careful manipulation and a learning curve is mandatory because increased experience results in a progressively higher success rate, less morbidity, shorter operating time, and fewer patients requiring open surgery.

Complications include perforation of the ureter, ureteric stricture, urinary leak following splitting of the intramural ureter, and a possible radiation hazard if the exposure time to fluoroscopy is too long.

51

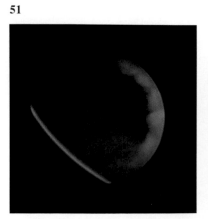

51 Open pelviureteric junction.

52

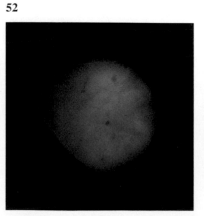

52 Inside renal pelvis.

53

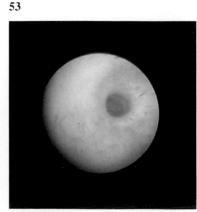

53 View into a calyx.

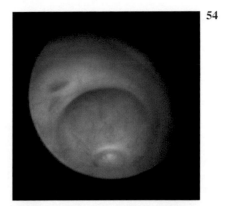

54 Duplicated ureter.

Ureteric stenting

Ureteric stents have revolutionised the management of stone disease with extracorporeal shockwave lithotripsy (ESWL) therapy, and their advent has removed the entity known as the stone street or *Steinstrasse*.

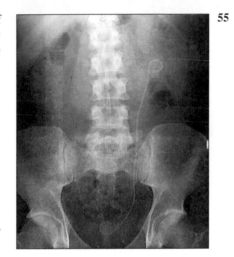

55 Left sided ureteric stent in position. (Double pigtail stent).

Conduitogram

The standard method of urinary diversion is the ileal conduit or 'Bricker Loop' technique. Radiological assessment of the upper tracts by IVU or conduitogram can be carried out.

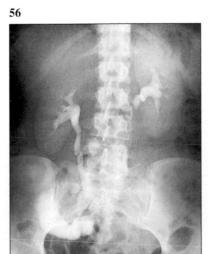

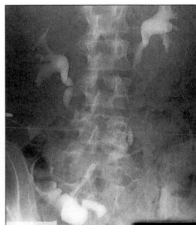

56 IVU of ileal conduit diversion shows normal upper tracts and outlines conduit.

57 Conduitogram. Full length film showing free reflux into both upper tracts and normal kidneys and ureters. The normal ureteroileal anastomosis is designed to allow free reflux and prevent stenosis.

Corpora cavernosography with pressure studies

The increased ability to investigate and manage the problems of impotence has resulted in the enhancement of radiological investigation by corpora cavernosography with associated pressure flow studies.

58

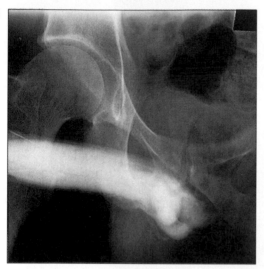

59

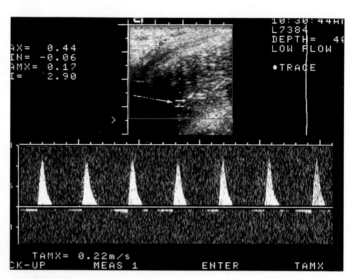

58 Normal corpora cavernosogram.

59 Normal papaverine stimulated penile Doppler ultrasound. The deep cavernosal arteries are identified by colour Doppler (arrow) and the spectral wave form measured. In this patient the maximum arterial flow in systole is 0.44 m/s with reversal of flow in diastole at -0.06 m/s.

Radionuclide renal scanning

Three types of renal scan are routinely performed in nuclear medicine:

- Dynamic renal scans.
- ^{99m}Tc DMSA (dimercaptosuccinic acid) static scans.
- Radionuclide cystography.

Dynamic renal scans

Three radiopharmaceuticals may be used: ^{99m}Tc DTPA (diethylenetriamine pentacetic acid), ^{99m}Tc MAG3, and ^{123}I-Hippuran. All give similar results and the choice of which to use depends on local factors such as cost and availability. The radiopharmaceutical is injected as a bolus and its transit through the kidneys is observed for 20–30 minutes. A background subtracted time–activity curve of each kidney is generated by the computer. This is the renogram curve. The early uptake phase allows accurate measurement of the differential function. In a kidney with impaired function the slope of this phase is reduced and the time to the peak lengthened. The third phase of the renogram curve reflects outflow tract function and can reveal either dilated outflow tracts or obstruction.

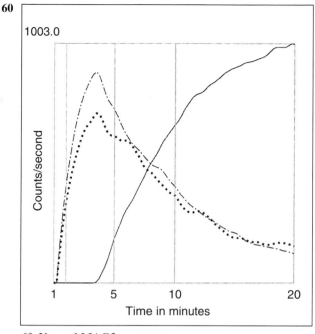

60

1003.0

Counts/second

Time in minutes

1   5   10   20

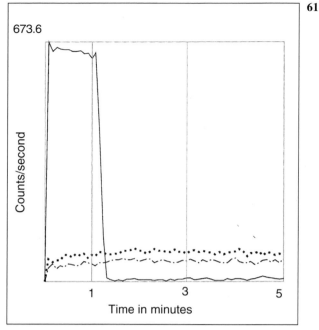

61

673.6

Counts/second

Time in minutes

1   3   5

60 Normal MAG3 renogram.
—·—·— = Left renogram*
············· = Right renogram*
———— = Bladder activity
Urinary flow rate = 5ml/minute

Relative Function
Left = 47%
Right = 53%
Volume voided =100ml

61 Normal MAG3 renogram voiding curves.
—·—·— = Left renogram*
············· = Right renogram*
———— = Bladder activity

*The curves are not normalised and are background subtracted.

62 Normal MAG3 isotope imaging at 5 minutes.

63 Normal MAG3 isotope imaging at 20 minutes.

62

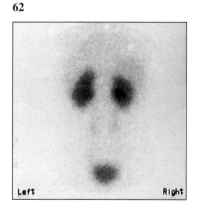

Left   Right

63

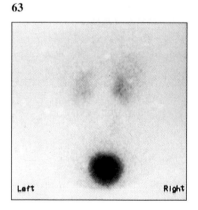

Left   Right

^{99m}Tc DMSA static scans

^{99m}Tc DMSA is taken up by the proximal tubular cells. Static images (posterior and oblique) are acquired 2 or 3 hours later. The relative uptake gives divided renal function. The main use for these scans is in the diagnosis of renal scarring, but they are also of use in the assessment of divided function, particularly in ectopic kidneys.

64

65

66

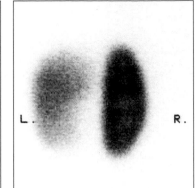

64 Normal ^{99m}Tc DMSA renal scan. Percentage glomerular filtration rate (GFR) – left 52, right 48. Left posterior oblique view.

65 Normal ^{99m}Tc DMSA renal scan. Percentage GFR – left 52, right 48. Posterior view.

66 Normal ^{99m}Tc DMSA renal scan. Length of kidney: left 8.8 cm, right 8.8 cm. Right posterior oblique view.

Radionuclide cystography

This can be performed either directly with an installation of ^{99m}Tc into the bladder via a catheter or indirectly following a dynamic renal scan. Its main use is to detect reflux and it is particularly useful in the follow-up assessment of such patients because the radiation dose to the patient is less than with radiological cystography (see **278**, p. 72).

67

Bone scan

Bone scans use ^{99m}Tc-labelled diphosphonates to localise sites of tumour involvement. Images are acquired using a gamma camera.

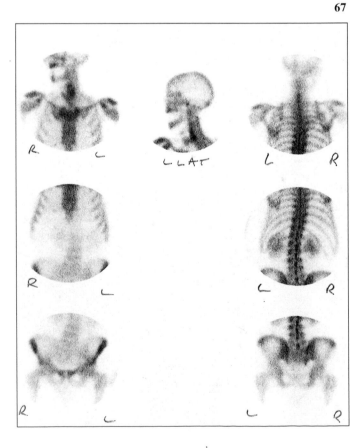

67 Normal bone scan.

The Whitaker test

The apparatus measures the pressure drop between the renal pelvis and the bladder and is another method of differentiating between an obstructive and a nonobstructive lesion in the urinary tract. A pressure drop of less than 10 cm of water at an injection rate of 10 ml/minute indicates no obstruction.

68

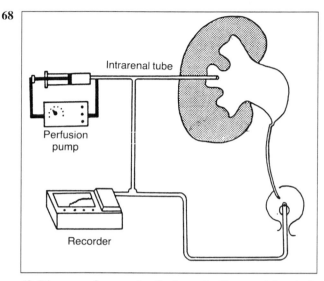

68 Diagram of apparatus for investigating a pelviureteric obstruction. Pressure is measured in the pelvis and the bladder at a perfusion of 10 ml/minute.

69

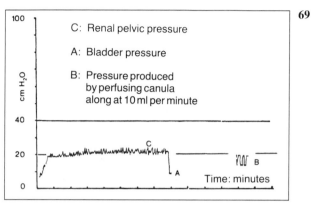

C: Renal pelvic pressure

A: Bladder pressure

B: Pressure produced by perfusing canula along at 10 ml per minute

69 Normal recording.

Blood supply of normal kidney

70 Normal kidney. A bisected normal kidney showing capsule, cortex, medulla, pelvis and ureter, pelvic fat, and vessels at the hilum (formalin fixed).

71 Cast of the venous drainage of a normal kidney.

70

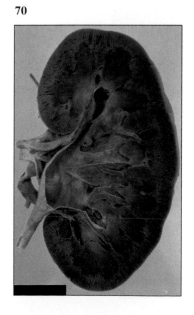

71

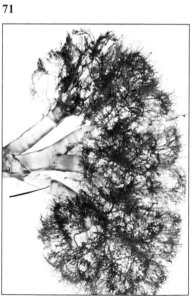

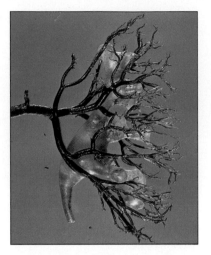

72 Blood supply cast. The main stem of the renal artery divides into the anterior and posterior division; the anterior division supplies four segments on the front of the kidney – the apical segment, the upper segment, the middle segment, and the lower segment. The posterior division continues into and becomes the artery to the posterior segment, which occupies a large central area on the back of the organ. In this cast, the divisions are so short that the anterior division of the renal artery almost divides into its segmental branches at one point.

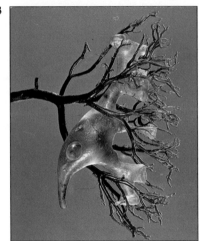

73 Posterior view of the same cast of the right kidney. The posterior division arises from the main stem of the renal artery to supply two-thirds of the renal substance on the posterior aspect of the organ. As it approaches the hilum, it becomes continuous with the artery of the posterior segment, which in turn divides into three sets of branches—an upper, a middle, and a terminal group. The area supplied by the last (and lowest) of these three vessels is adjacent to and above the territory of the posterior branch of the lower segment artery (branch of the anterior division).

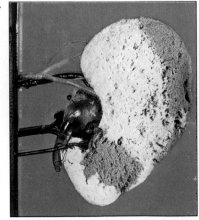

74 Renal arterial supply by multiple vessels. Some kidneys are supplied by multiple arteries. This cast shows a kidney seen from behind and supplied by three segmental arteries, each of which has arisen directly from the aorta. Each artery was injected with a resin of a different colour. The apical segmental and the posterior segmental arteries are in yellow resin, which has become off-white because of the colour dilution in the finer vessels of the cortex. The anterior division supplying the upper and middle segments is in red resin. The anterior branch of the lower segment artery is in blue and the posterior branch of the lower segment artery is in red.

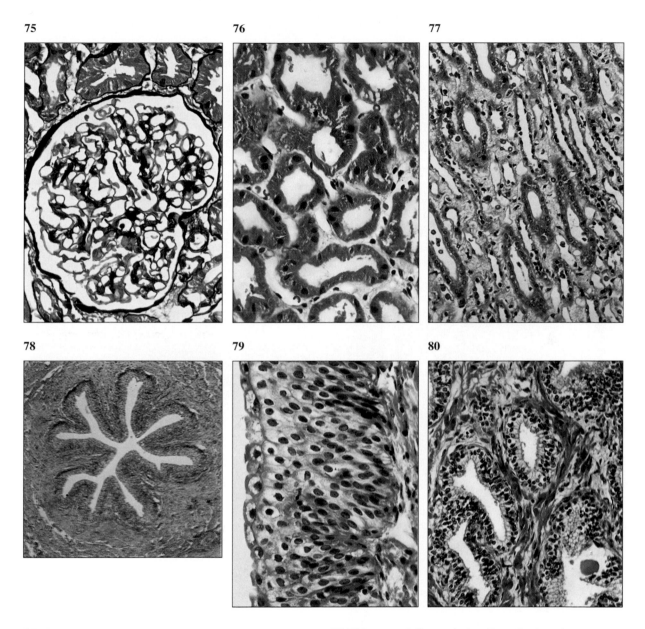

75   **Normal glomerulus.** Section through a glomerulus showing the hilum at the right of the field. Bowman's capsule surrounds the urinary space within which is the glomerular tuft. This is made up of capillaries communicating with the afferent and efferent arterioles at the hilum. In the tuft the methenamine silver picks up the basement membrane and mesangial matrix. The capillaries are open and the urinary filtrate is formed across the basement membrane (with its endothelial and epithelial cells) into the urinary space. *(Methenamine silver x 256)*

76   **Kidney: cortical tubules.** The proximal and distal convoluted tubules are situated in the cortex and modify the glomerular filtrate. *(H&E x 256)*

77   **Kidney: medullary tubules.** The collecting tubules and the loops of Henle are seen in the medulla. *(H&E x 160)*

78   **Ureter.** This is lined with transitional epithelium. There is a little subepithelial connective tissue and then the muscle coats—an inner longitudinal layer and an outer circular layer with a second longitudinal layer in the lower third. The adventitia is outside the muscle. *(H&E x 26)*

79   **Transitional epithelium lines the urothelial tract from the renal pelvis to the urethra.** It is a multilayered epithelium, normally up to about seven layers thick. The most superficial cells are wider and cover a few underlying cells. This section is from a ureter. *(H&E x 256)*

80   **Prostate.** Normal prostatic glands in fibromuscular stroma. *(H&E x 160)*

81

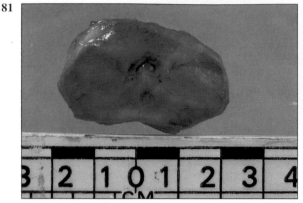

81 Prostate showing normal-sized lobes and urethra from a 24-year-old male who died from unrelated lesions.

82

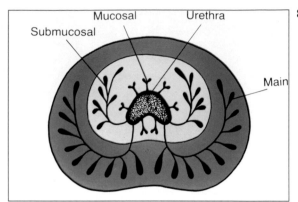

82 Diagram of duct system of the lobes of the prostate.

83

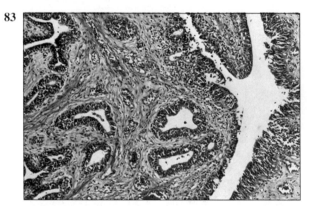

83 Urethra and verumontanum. Prostatic ducts opening on verumontanum into the urethra on the right of the field. *(H&E x 64)*

84

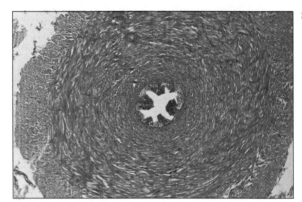

84 Vas deferens. This duct is lined by columnar, pseudo-stratified epithelium and surrounded by three muscle coats – an inner and an outer longitudinal, and a middle circular layer. *(H&E x 16)*

85

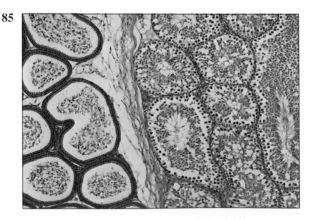

85 Testis and epididymis. Testicular tubules on the right-hand side of the field; epididymal tubules on the left. The testis is a compound tubular gland divided into over 200 components and surrounded by a fibrous capsule, the tunica albuginea. These components consist of seminiferous tubules which show spermatogenesis with spermatozoa in various stages of maturation. Sertoli cells, which are attached to the basement membrane, are also seen. The interstitial tissue consists of connective tissue, blood, and lymph vessels, a few cells and the cells of Leydig (see also **1333** and **1334**). The seminiferous tubules pass into the rete testis and form the ducti efferentes, which pass through the head, body, and tail of the epididymis to form the vas deferens. In the proximal part of the epididymis the lumen is lined by pseudostratified columnar epithelium, but the cells disappear as the ductus epididymis approaches the globus minor.

86

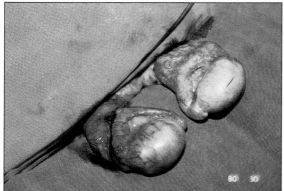

86 Testes and epididymes.

87

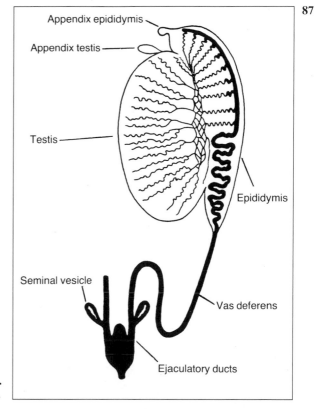

Appendix epididymis

Appendix testis

Testis

Epididymis

Seminal vesicle

Vas deferens

Ejaculatory ducts

87 Diagram of testis and duct system.
(See also testicular ultrasound on pp 12–13).

Crystals

● **Amorphous phosphates.** Fine granular forms, often found in urine that has been standing for some time. May be mistaken for bacteria by the inexperienced microscopist.

● **Calcium oxalate**—'envelope' crystals.
● **Triple phosphates** (ammonium magnesium phosphate) – 'coffin-lid' crystals of varying size.

Crystals in the urine

88

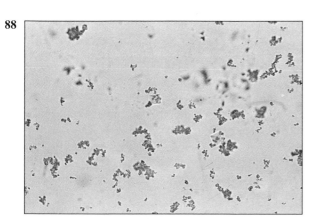

88 Amorphous phosphates.

89

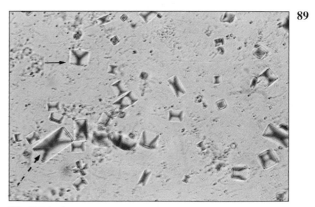

89 Calcium oxalate (arrow) and triple phosphate (dotted arrow).

90

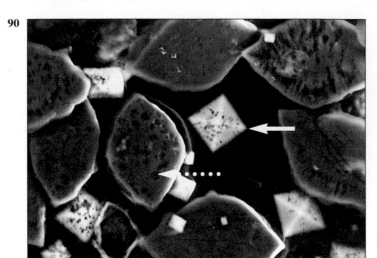

90 Scanning electron microscopy of oxalate (arrow) and uric acid crystals (dotted arrow).

Haematology

Dysmorphic red cells.

91

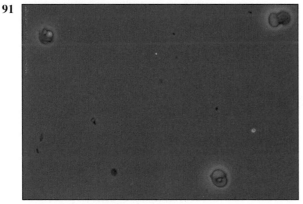

Haematuria of renal origin often shows a high proportion of dysmorphic red cells on phase contrast microscopy. These red cells show small blebs on their surface membranes. Urine for this investigation should be examined fresh: after a few hours red cells may become artefactually dysmorphic.

91 Urine: phase contrast microscopy with additional green filter.

Sickle-cell disease

92

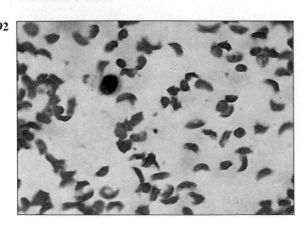

Haemoglobinopathy is seen in negroid races. The abnormality is that one amino acid, glutamic acid, is substituted by valine in the sixth position of the amino acid chain of haemoglobin under reduced oxygen tension. This causes it to become less soluble and to crystallise out, producing the classic sickle-shaped red cells, shown in **92**, which may lead to haematuria and produce renal lesions.

92 Classic sickle-shaped red cells. *(Giemsa)*

Endoscopy

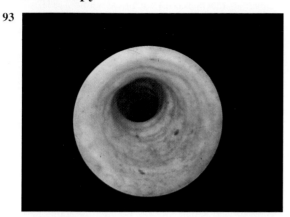

93 Anterior urethra showing vascular pattern, which in this part of the urethra is irregular.

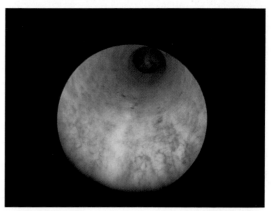

94 Bulbar urethra showing change in the vascular pattern, a greater number of vessels are present, and they are conforming to a more longitudinal arrangement.

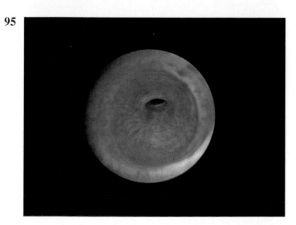

95 Membranous urethra. The vessels now run long-itudinally and converge towards the external sphincter.

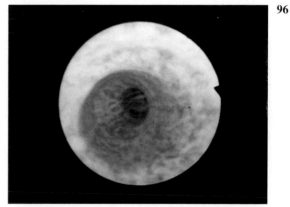

96 The membranous urethra seen through a flexible cystoscope.

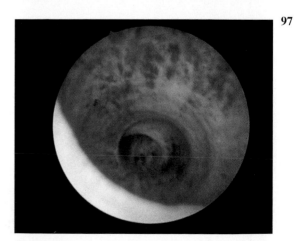

97 The same view seen through the rigid instrument.

98

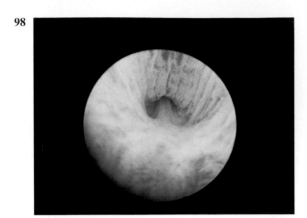

98 External sphincter. The circular pattern is clearly seen. In the prostatic urethra there is a median ridge called the urethral crest, which extends from the bladder neck to the external sphincter caused by elevation of the mucous membrane and the underlying tissue. In the middle of the crest is the colliculus seminalis or verumontanum, on the tip of which open the ejaculatory ducts. On either side of the crest there is a depression into which the prostatic ducts open.

99

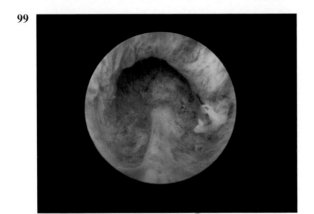

99 A normal urethral crest.

100

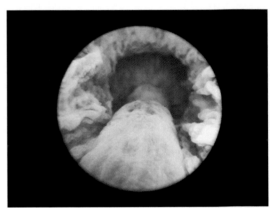

100 Verumontanum with the opening of the ejaculatory ducts clearly visible on the dome.

101

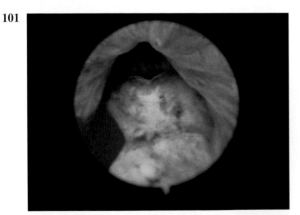

101 Lobulated verumontanum. A variant of the normal, but one which is liable to give rise to terminal haematuria.

102

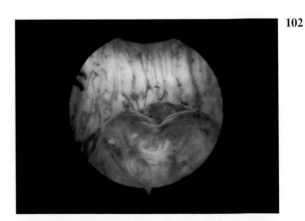

102 A more pronounced lobulation of the verumontanum.

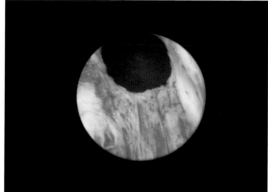

103 Normal bladder neck in a young male. The margins are smooth with a pronounced vascular pattern.

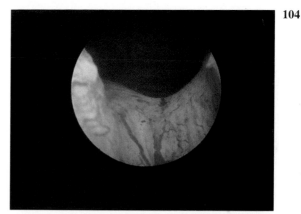

104 Normal bladder neck in a middle-aged male. The margins may be irregular and slight enlargement of the right lateral lobe of the prostate is visible.

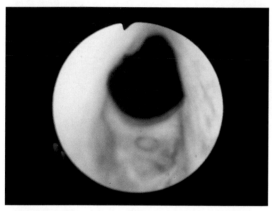

105 A similar view to that shown in 104 as seen through the flexible cystoscope.

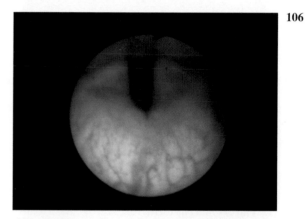

106 Bladder neck and slightly enlarged prostate in front of it as seen through the flexible cystoscope.

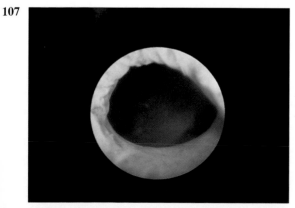

107 Normal bladder neck in a young female. The outline is smooth and merges posteriorly into the base of the bladder.

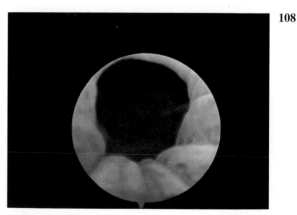

108 Normal bladder neck in a post-menopausal female. The mucous membrane is oedematous, more vascular, and arranged in folds.

109
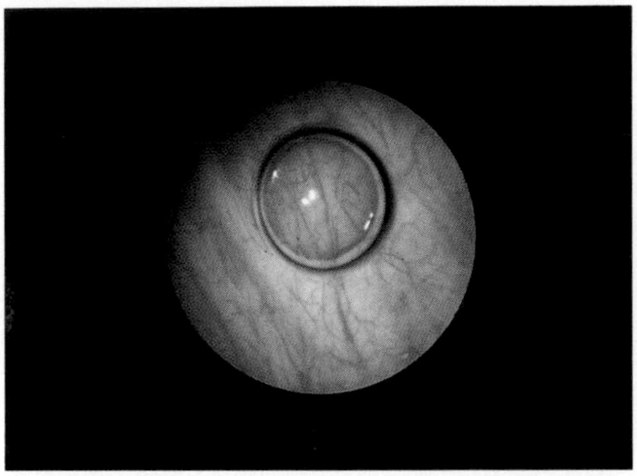

109 Air bubble, at the bladder fundus. An excellent initial landmark for the inexperienced urologist.

110
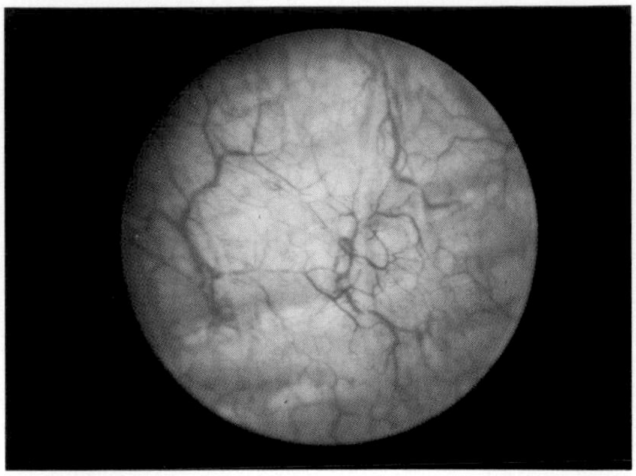

110 Normal bladder vessels.

111
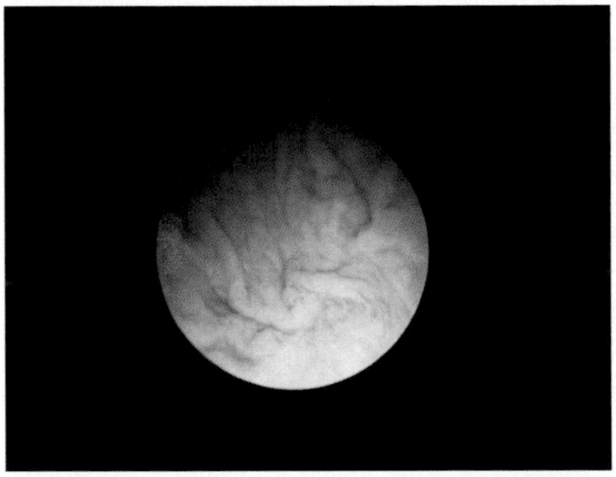

111 Flaccid mucous membrane. The normal appearance of the bladder before it is distended with fluid.

112
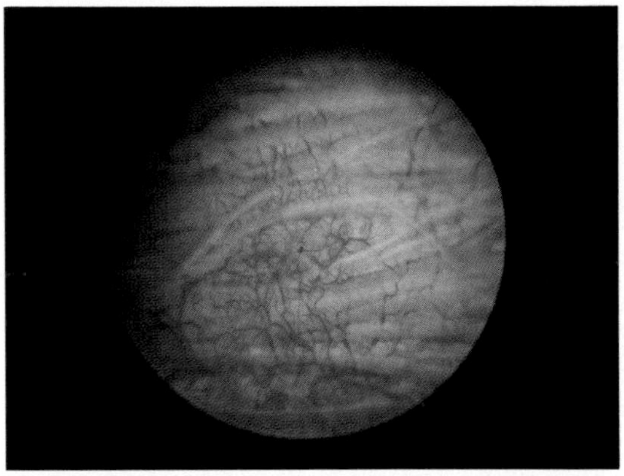

112 Normal bladder muscle. There is no set pattern. The individual muscle bundles appear as discrete strands, which can be distinctly separated from each other.

113
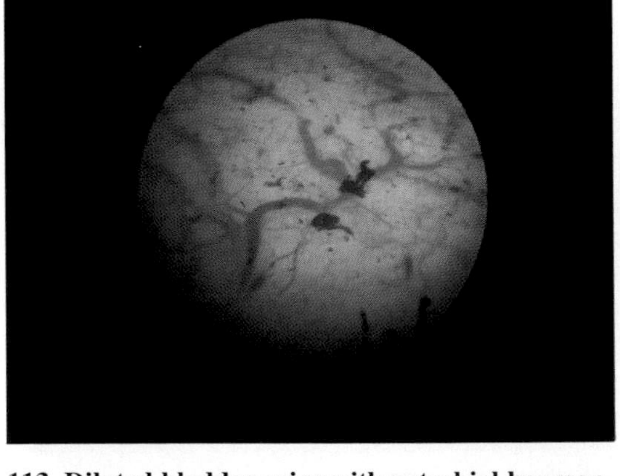

113 Dilated bladder veins with petechial haemorrhages. The normal appearance of the bladder after it is distended with fluid.

Variations of the normal ureteric orifice

The final stages of development of the ureteric orifices are complex. The connection between the ureter and the bladder is brought about through Waldeyer's muscle sheath, which has a lateral and medial component, both of which separate in the bladder to form different parts of the trigone. It is therefore not surprising that the normal ureteric orifice shows many variations.

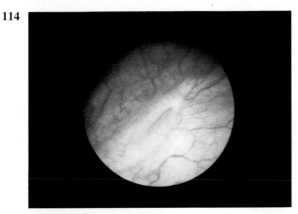

114 The slit type of orifice.

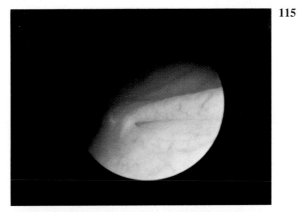

115 Orifice on outer side of ureteric bar.

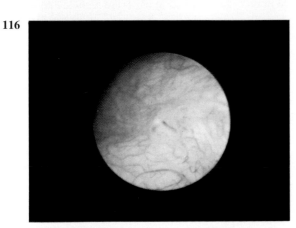

116 Shallow orifice with no ureteric bar.

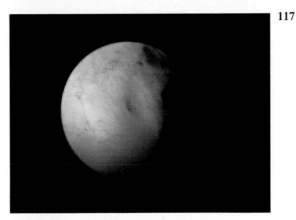

117 Orifice on top of a mound.

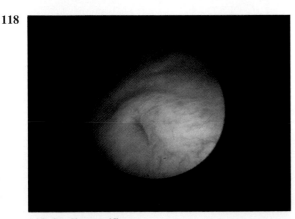

118 Stadium orifice.

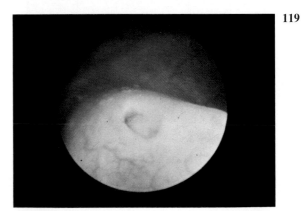

119 Flat crescentic orifice.

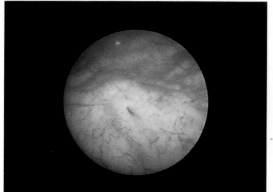

120 Orifice with mild trabeculation.

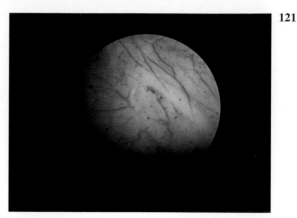

121 Orifice which appears withdrawn and contracted.

Urodynamics

Videocystometrogram

The patient is catheterised with either a double-lumen catheter or two catheters – the larger, through which the bladder is filled, is removed before micturition, the smaller measures bladder pressure. A further catheter in the rectum monitors abdominal pressure, which can be subtracted from bladder pressure to give the true (intrinsic) bladder pressure. Males stand at, and females sit on, a commode beneath which a flow meter monitors the volume of urine passed and automatically computes the flow rate in ml/s (122). All parameters are recorded on a multichannel recorder and the chart viewed with a TV camera (123). The bladder is filled with contrast medium and viewed with an X-ray unit mounted on a 'C' arm for mobility (124). A split TV screen shows synchronously the measured parameters and cystogram image, and can be recorded on videotape. Electromyography (EMG) of the external sphincters can also be recorded.

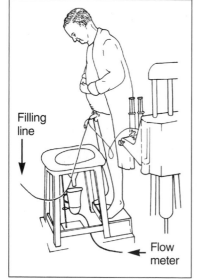

122 Male patient undergoing pressure–flow studies.

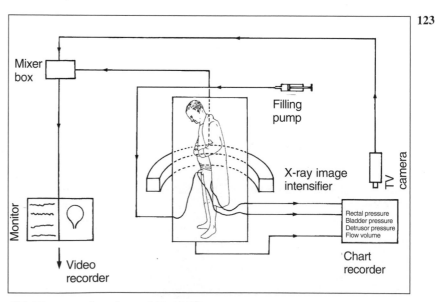

123 Diagram of urodynamic apparatus.

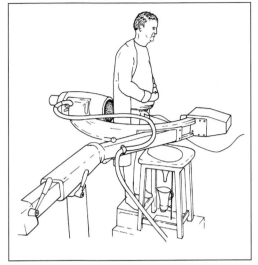

124 Male patient prepared for videocystometrogram with image intensifier in place.

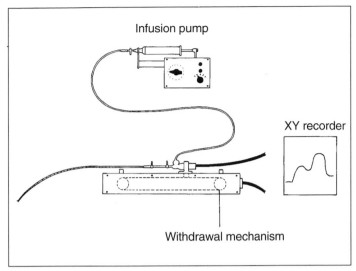

125 Urethral pressure profile equipment. A special catheter with a closed end and a rosette of subterminal openings is placed in the bladder. Fluid is slowly infused by means of a constant flow pump. The catheter is mechanically withdrawn at a constant rate. The pressure within the catheter is recorded and a profile of the static pressure conditions along the length of the urethra is obtained. The patient can also be asked to contract the external sphincter to observe the alteration in the profile.

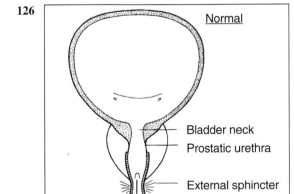

126 Normal male bladder and urethra during micturition.

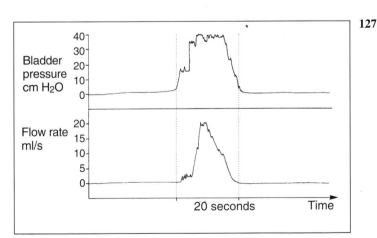

127 Pressure–flow study of normal micturition. In the normal bladder, filling results in a small pressure rise to the point of fullness. Micturition is under voluntary control and accomplished by a smooth increase in intravesical pressure. Because detrusor fibres are inserted in the proximal urethra, the bladder neck is pulled open. The external sphincter relaxes coincidentally.

128

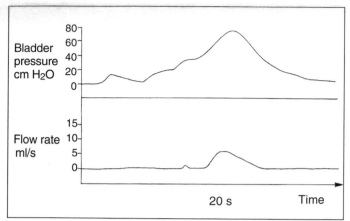

129

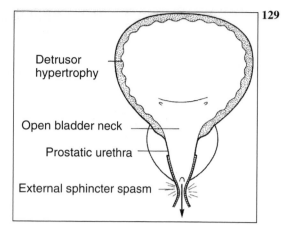

128 Pressure–flow study of detrusor instability. Involuntary uninhibited detrusor contractions occur as a result of overt neurological disease representing an upper-motor neurone lesion or may be seen as an idiopathic phenomenon. These contractions can cause frequency, urgency, or frank incontinence. Alternatively lower-motor neurone lesions result in low pressure 'autonomic' detrusor contractions and ineffective bladder emptying.

129 Spastic external sphincter.

130

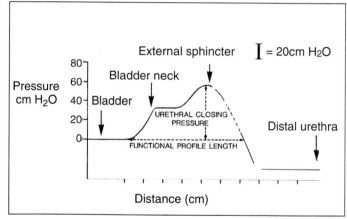

130 Diagrammatic representation of normal male urethral pressure profile.

131

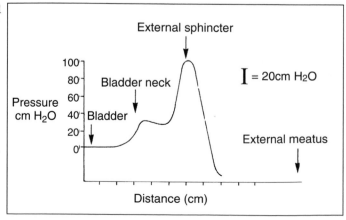

131 Urethral pressure profile: external sphincter spasm.

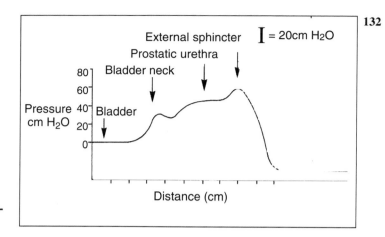

132 Urethral pressure profile: prostatic obstruction.

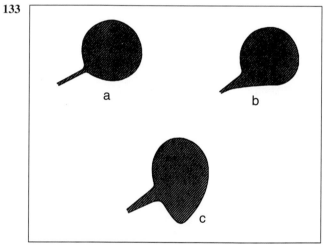

133 Video appearances of lateral view of female bladder on coughing. Weakness of the female pelvic floor causes variable descent of the bladder base and proximal urethra; stress incontinence results when neck region support is poor. (a = normal, b = stress incontinence, c = stress incontinence with marked cystocele)

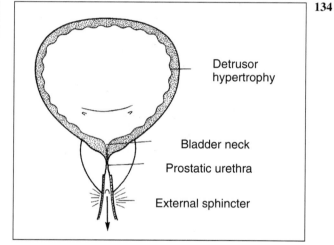

134 Prostatic obstruction.

Vesicoureteric reflux may be primary or secondary to outflow tract obstruction, with or without neurological bladder disease. Video/pressure/flow studies aid full assessment and diagnosis.

135

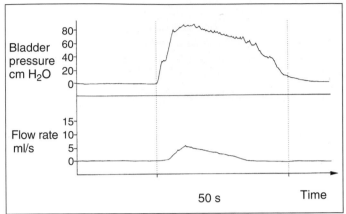

135 Pressure–flow study of prostatic obstruction. This trace shows the high bladder pressure and poor flow rate in prostatic obstruction. Outflow obstruction produced by bladder neck hypertrophy or prostatic intrusion into the urethra results in detrusor hypertrophy with high pressure contractions, low flow rate, and poor opening of the neck or proximal urethra during micturition.

136

```
50 ml/s Flow Rate
```

Results of Uroflowmetry		
Voiding time	T100	14 s
Flow time	TQ	13 s
Time to max. flow	TQmax	6 s
Max. flow rate	Qmax	34.9 ml/s
Average flow rate	Qave	15.9 ml/s
Voided volume	Vcomp	210 ml

136 Normal urinary flow pattern. The shape of the flow pattern is significant and, when it becomes flattened, prolonged and intermittent, it indicates outflow obstruction. Maximum flows under 20ml/s are abnormal. This noninvasive and easily performed test can be used to monitor progress following all methods of treatment.

2 Congenital abnormalities

The routine use of ultrasound investigation in pregnancy has resulted in antenatal detection of most congenital abnormalities. Fetal hydronephrosis is very common (1 in 200 pregnancies) and is not always synonymous with pathology; the fetal glomerular filtration rate is higher than that of the infant, and in some cases fetal hydronephrosis disappears after birth. It is also important to remember that ultrasound gives no functional information and that the current methods of assessing renal function before birth are very crude i.e. noting the presence of oligohydramnios (indicating obstructive uropathy or bilateral renal disease) or direct needle puncture of the hydronephrotic kidney and biochemical analysis of the urine obtained.

Presenting symptoms

Congenital abnormalities may be detected in asymptomatic individuals of any age. In the fetus the normal bladder should be visible by 14 weeks of gestation, and the normal kidneys should be visible by 15–18 weeks of gestation (several weeks after the onset of fetal urine production) with routine antenatal ultrasound examination. In the infant or child abnormalities may be revealed during routine screening investigations for other diseases (e.g. congenital cardiac anomalies). The non-invasive nature of ultrasound has resulted in its use to investigate a number of abdominal and pelvic disorders, and the chance finding of asymptomatic urinary tract pathology is becoming more common in adults.

When congenital abnormalities do produce symptoms, they usually consist of abdominal pain, urinary tract infection, haematuria, or voiding difficulties, and many individuals do not develop symptoms until adult life. Investigation of symptomatic or asymptomatic hypertension, may uncover congenital urinary tract pathology. Congenital hydronephrosis may present for the first time following relatively minor trauma because the susceptibility to injury is greater than normal.

Urinary tract abnormalities detected by antenatal ultrasound examination

Ultrasound can detect an absent fetal kidney or bladder, and can provide limited information about bladder size and its ability to empty. It can also reveal hydronephrosis and oligohydramnios, but can not distinguish between obstructive and nonobstructive uropathy, and the precise diagnosis is not possible until after birth, when functional imaging and cystography can be performed.

The combination of bilateral hydronephrosis and oligohydramnios during the second trimester is usually fatal due to severe pulmonary hypoplasia, irrespective of the exact diagnosis. There is as yet no evidence that antenatal decompression of the urinary tract or early elective delivery improves the prognosis of these cases. Currently the main advantage of antenatal ultrasound is to alert the clinician to the presence of urinary tract pathology so that prompt diagnosis and treatment takes place immediately after birth before symptoms develop.

The following conditions may be detected antenatally, with diagnosis made postnatally:

- Pelviureteric junction (PUJ) obstruction (unilateral or bilateral).
- Multicystic kidney.
- Infantile polycystic kidneys.
- Renal agenesis.
- Megaureter (obstructive or nonobstructive).
- Ectopic ureterocele or ureter.
- Vesicoureteric reflux.
- Bladder exstrophy.
- Posterior urethral valves.
- Prune belly syndrome.
- Urethral atresia.

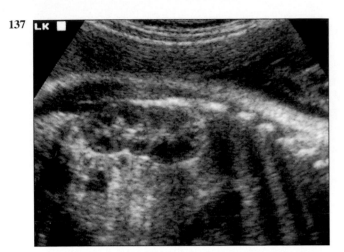

137 Antenatal ultrasound scan at 16 weeks showing normal left kidney.

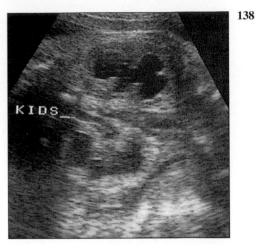

138 Antenatal ultrasound scan at 16 weeks showing bilateral hydronephrosis.

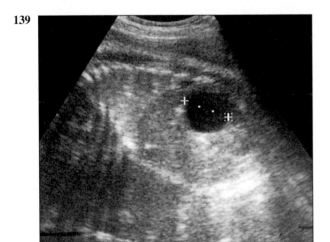

139 Antenatal ultrasound scan at 18 weeks showing unilateral ? renal cyst ? hydronephrosis (could be a duplex).

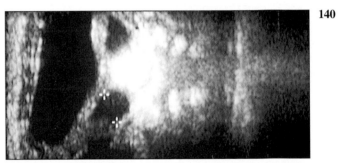

140 Antenatal ultrasound scan showing bilateral ureteric dilatation (normal ureters are not usually detectable).

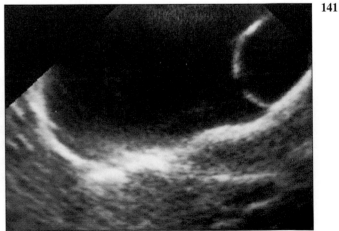

141 Antenatal ultrasound scan at 20 weeks showing ureterocele in the bladder.

142 Diagram of the developing urinary system up to the fourth week (adapted from numerous sources). At the fourth week the pronephros has almost completely disappeared, while mesonephric tubules have begun to form in the mesonephric duct. At this stage the earliest signs of the ureteric bud can be seen arising from the mesonephric tissue.

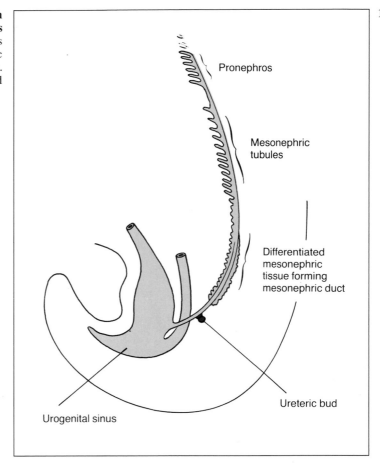

Pronephros

Mesonephric tubules

Differentiated mesonephric tissue forming mesonephric duct

Ureteric bud

Urogenital sinus

Abnormalities of the kidneys

Anomalies of number

For the kidney to develop properly a normal ureteric bud must penetrate a normal metanephric blastema between 5–7 weeks of gestation.

An absent kidney is due to failure of the ureteric bud, and if any portion of ureter exists, there is usually a small associated kidney. An absent hemitrigone at cystoscopy indicates unilateral renal agenesis. Unilateral renal agenesis in girls is associated with partial or complete nonunion of the müllerian duct system. Bilateral renal agenesis occurs in 1 in 4000 fetuses and is associated with anhydramnios.

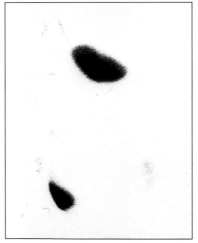

143

143 Absent kidney. DMSA scan shows no function in the right kidney.

144

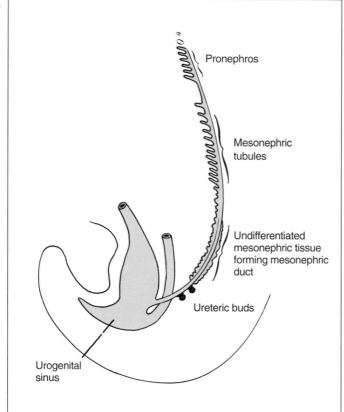

Pronephros

Mesonephric
tubules

Undifferentiated
mesonephric tissue
forming mesonephric
duct

Ureteric buds

Urogenital
sinus

144 Embryological diagram of embryo at four weeks showing two ureteric buds. Ureteric anomalies account for about 30% of all congenital abnormalities in the urinary tract; up to 10% of all patients seen at urological clinics have some ureteric abnormality. The duplication of the ureter is caused by either early branching of the ascending ureter and its extent depends on the time when the ureter branches, or the second ureteric bud, which arises from the mesonephric duct. This diagram, which is only a very little older than the first, shows two ureteric buds and this is the cause of a duplication in the urinary tract.

145

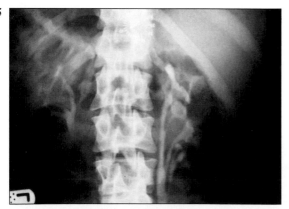

145 Bifid kidney. The division is in the upper third of the ureter and is caused by late branching of the ureteric ampulla. This condition can give rise to abnormal peristalis in the ureter leading to the 'yo-yo' flow of urine from one moiety to the other.

146

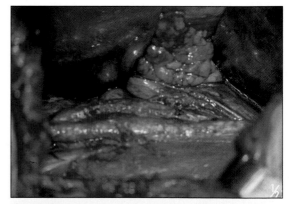

146 Duplex system starting at the upper third of the ureter indicative of late branching.

147 Upper third duplex system with the drooping lily appearance of the opposite side.

148 Duplex system in which the two systems join in the middle third of the ureter indicating earlier branching of the ureteric bud.

147

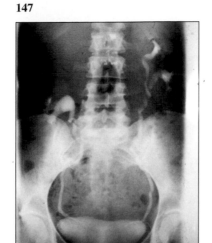

148

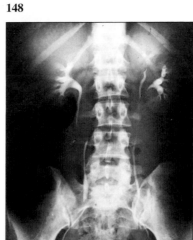

149 Lower third ureteric duplication with one small kidney moiety.

150 Retrograde pyelogram of lower third ureteric duplication in which one ureter opens into an ectopic hypoplastic kidney as a result of failure of development of one of the duplicated ureters.

149

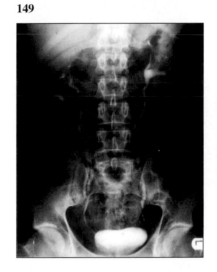

150

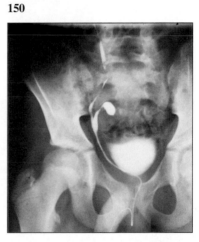

151

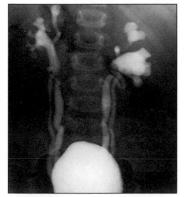

151 Complete duplex.

152

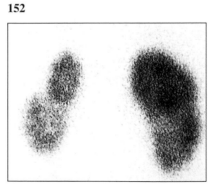

152 DMSA scan showing bilateral duplex systems. A scan may sometimes demonstrate duplex more clearly than an IVU.

153

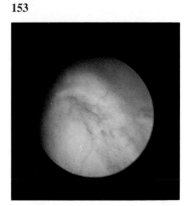

153 Duplex ureteric orifices. The upper orifice is always from the lower moiety. The hooded type is the one most likely to reflux.

Abnormalities of position

Ascent of the kidney is complete by 8 weeks of gestation.

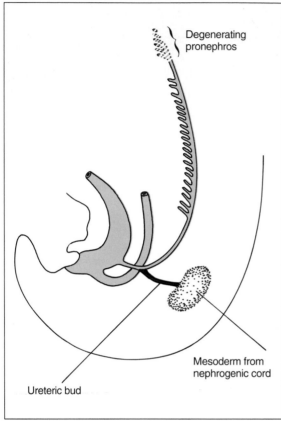

154 Embryological diagram of embryo at 6 weeks. The pronephros is degenerating and the ureteric bud has now joined the mesoderm from the nephrogenic cord; the mesonephric duct moves caudally to be absorbed into the vesicourethral area.

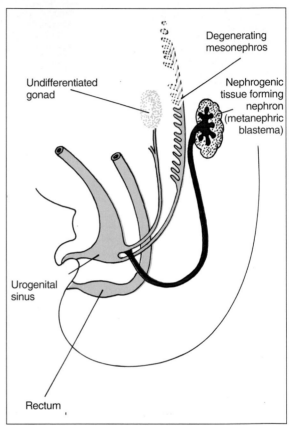

155 Embryological diagram of embryo at 8 weeks. At this time the cloaca has differentiated into the urinary and lower bowel systems. The ureter, with its cap of mesoderm, has moved caudally and the undifferentiated gonads are first seen. Malrotation is not an uncommon finding. The calyces usually point vertically rather than laterally. The condition rarely causes any problem.

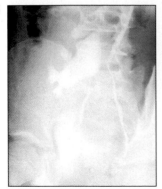

156 Unilateral pelvic ectopic kidney. PUJ obstruction and stones are common.

157 MAG3 scan of pelvic kidney with contralateral duplex.

158

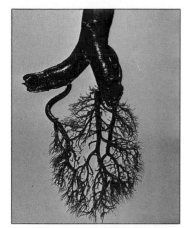

158 Blood supply of ectopic kidney lying in the hollow of the skeletal pelvis. It is supplied by three arteries, which bear no relationship to the pattern found in either normal or congenitally abnormal kidneys in the lumbar region. In this cast, the kidney was supplied by three arteries, two of which shared a common origin from the bifurcation of the aorta, while the third arose from the left common iliac artery. However, the blood supply of any pelvic ectopic kidney is very small.

It is not known whether the thoracic kidney is due to ascent of the kidney before diaphragmatic closure, or whether there is a primary diaphragmatic defect enhancing renal ascent.

159

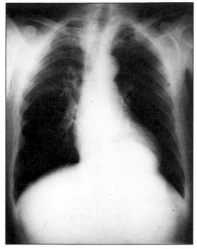

159 A thoracic kidney showing an abnormality of ascent. This shows the diaphragmatic defect.

161

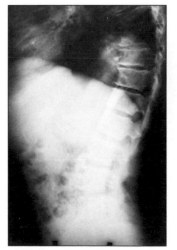

161 Lateral view of thoracic kidney.

160

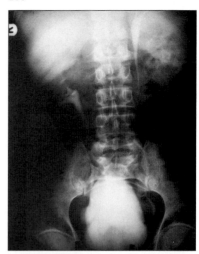

160 IVU showing left thoracic kidney in anteroposterior view.

162

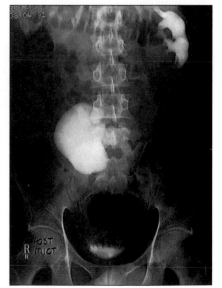

162 Bilateral malrotation.

Anomalies of position and fusion

Fusion is usually in the lower poles. The cause of this is probably an abnormality in ascent combined with some vascular abnormality, which leads to the lower poles failing to migrate laterally.

Horseshoe kidney

Occurs in 1 in 400 live births. The union is at the lower pole and a bridge of renal tissue crosses in front of the aorta, spine, and inferior vena cava. The long axes are parallel to the spine and there is an associated malrotation, the renal pelves lying anterior with the calyces posteriorly, laterally, or medially.

A characteristic feature which is pathognomonic of a horseshoe kidney is the medially directed lower calyces passing to the bridge of renal tissue. The unusual relation of the renal vessels sometimes leads to obstruction, which results in infection, hydronephrosis, or occasionally stone formation, or a combination of all three.

163

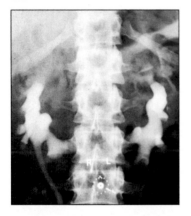

164

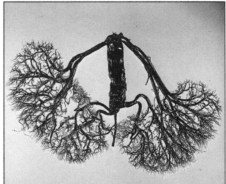

163 The horseshoe kidney is the commonest variety of renal fusion.

164 Blood supply of horseshoe kidney. The arteries to the apical, upper middle posterior segments on either side of the aorta are of the same pattern as those of normal kidneys. The right lower segmental arteries, however, have not only arisen from a common trunk, but the posterior branches of these vessels have arisen earlier than the anterior branches and almost directly from the aorta.

165

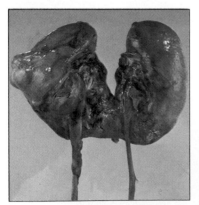

165 Horseshoe kidney. Here the lower poles are fused across the mid-line and the ureters pass down anteriorly.

166

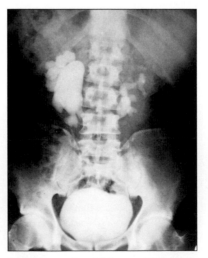

166 Horseshoe kidney with hydronephrosis of one kidney caused by ureteric obstruction usually at the pelviureteric junction.

167

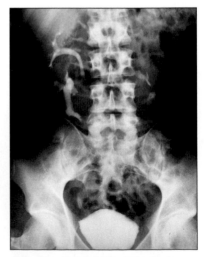

167 Horseshoe kidney in the lower pole of a bilateral duplex system, the upper moiety on the left side having been removed.

Complications of horseshoe kidney

168 Ureteric reflux. Vesicoureteric reflux into the left half of a horseshoe kidney.

169 Resected specimen showing dilated pelvis and diminished renal parenchyma due to persistent reflux and chronic recurrent infection.

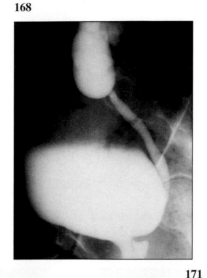

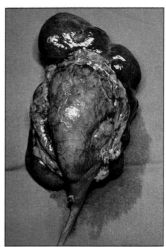

Crossed ectopia

170 Crossed ectopia with fusion. Crossed ectopia of one kidney fused with the other kidney with only one pelvicalyceal system.

171 Crossed ectopia without fusion. Two separate crossed ectopic kidneys with separate pelvicalyceal systems.

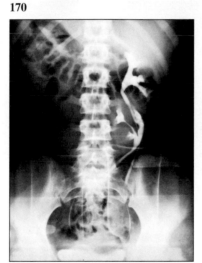

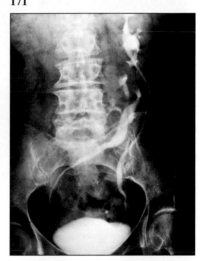

Anomalies of structure

Multicystic–dysplastic disease

This can be diagnosed *in utero*.

172 Histology of multicystic–dysplastic kidney with adrenal gland above, removed soon after birth. Although most multicystic-dysplastic kidneys involve during infancy, it is thought, but by no means proven, that they should be removed because of the possibility of later malignancy.

173 Ultrasound scan of the same kidney before birth. In the absence of a kidney it is easy to see how the adrenal gland may be mistaken for renal tissue on antenatal ultrasound examination.

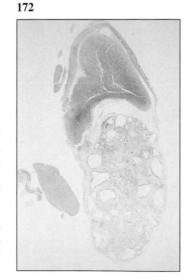

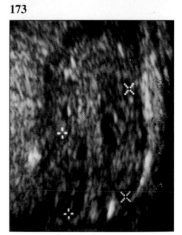

174

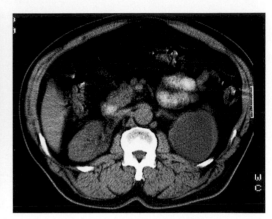

175

174 IVU showing a left multicystic kidney with calyceal displacement.

175 CT scan of a left multicystic kidney.

176

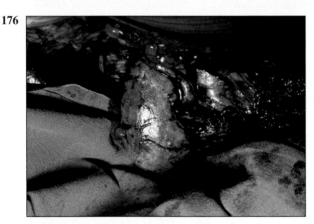

177

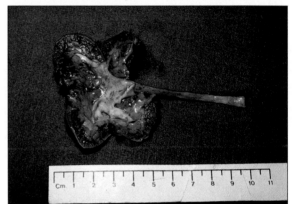

176 Hypoplastic kidney before nephrectomy. The kidney is small and of normal colour and shape.

177 Hypoplastic kidney. Section of the same kidney showing thin cortex and very little functioning renal tissue. This kidney was discovered on routine examination for essential hypertension.

178

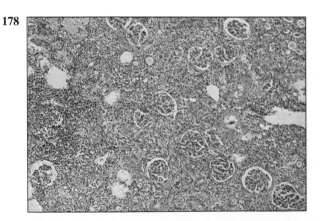

179

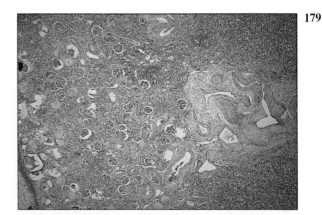

178, 179 Hypoplastic kidney. Histology of the same kidney. The sections show atrophy of the tubules, a heavy chronic inflammatory cell infiltrate in the interstitium, and hypertensive changes in the vessels. These changes, together with the dilatation of some tubules and focal calcification, may be secondary.

180 Dysplastic kidney. This kidney is an example of the group of disorders in which abnormal metanephric differentiation is seen, frequently associated with cyst formation. The abnormal structures are recognised histologically (see **181** and **182**). Most cases described as aplastic, hypoplastic, or multicystic kidney are really variants of this disorder.

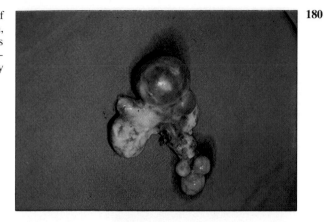

180

181, 182 Dysplastic kidney. The pictures show an abnormal renal parenchyma with a paucity of nephrons. The abnormal ducts and tubules, lined by cuboidal to columnar epithelium, which is sometimes ciliated are surrounded by cellular mesenchyme. Cartilage is sometimes present. The cysts are lined by flat epithelium.

181

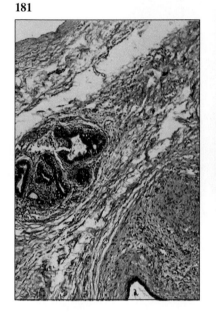

182

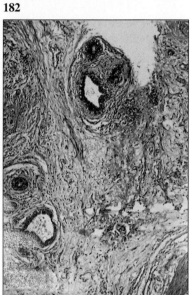

Polycystic disease

Polycystic disease occurs in two major forms. Both have a hereditary basis and both involve all parts of both kidneys. The adult type (autosomal dominant, though many are new mutations) usually presents in adult life with hypertension and renal failure or haematuria. The kidneys are often massively enlarged. The infantile form (autosomal recessive) gives rise to kidneys that cannot support life, and death occurs early.

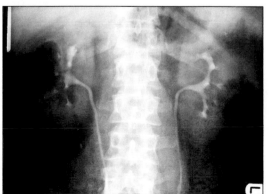

183

183 Example of polycystic disease.

184

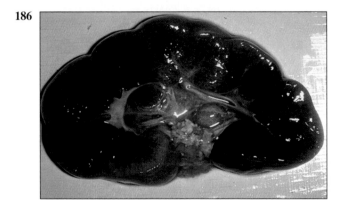

184 Ultrasound showing polycystic kidneys.

186

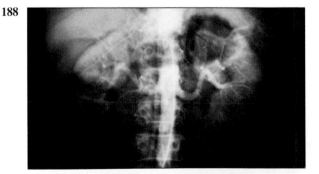

186 Infantile polycystic kidneys. This form of polycystic disease results in kidneys that cannot support life. Cystically dilated tubules radiate from the pelvis to the cortex. This specimen came from an infant who died within 2 days of birth.

188

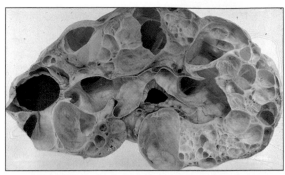

188 Arteriogram showing the avascular upper pole caused by the cyst and the tumour blush in the tumour.

185

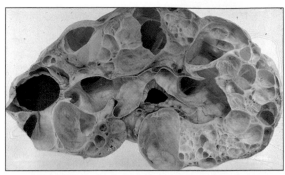

185 Adult type polycystic kidney. This is a formalin-fixed specimen from a postmortem of a young adult dying of cerebral haemorrhage associated with hypertension. Both kidneys were like this one. They are very much larger than the infantile polycystic kidney.

187

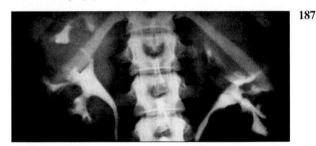

187 IVU of a polycystic kidney in which a carcinoma has developed on the lower pole distorting the calyces and the pelvis.

189

190

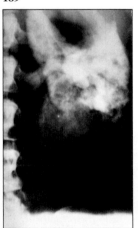

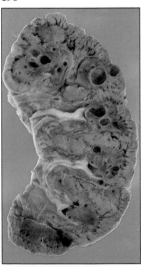

189 Arteriogram – nephrogram phase. This confirms a lower pole tumour.

190 Medullary sponge kidney. There are multiple small cysts in the medulla and a little scarring of the cortex. Possibly caused by secondary infection, it was an incidental finding at postmortem of an elderly lady who died from an unrelated disease.

Abnormalities of the collecting system

191

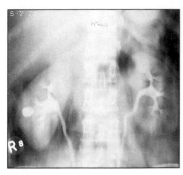

191 Plain abdominal X-ray and IVU showing large calyceal calculus producing minimal renal damage. This is a stone within a calyceal cyst.

192

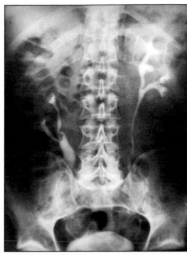

193

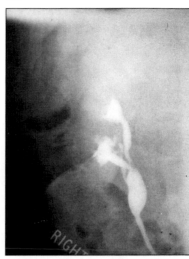

192, 193 A very unusual abnormality of formation of the pelvicalyceal system showing a blind calyx coming off from the front of the pelvis. Ultrasonography and arteriography failed to show any renal substance attached to this single calyceal stem, so it must be assumed that it is a blind calyceal bud that has failed to join up with any renal parenchyma.

Pelviureteric junction (PUJ) obstruction

PUJ obstruction is a common intermittent partial obstruction of the collecting system. Usually it is asymptomatic until puberty, but may remain asymptomatic throughout life, or may even present with pyonephrosis in old age.

Diagnosis before symptoms occur as a result of antenatal ultrasound poses a dilemma as to which patients need treatment because the natural history of the disorder is unknown.

194

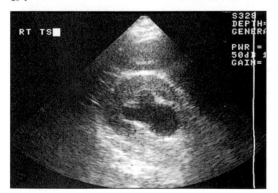

194 Ultrasound showing unilateral hydronephrosis, the most common cause being PUJ obstruction.

195 IVU showing bilateral PUJ obstruction in an infant.

195

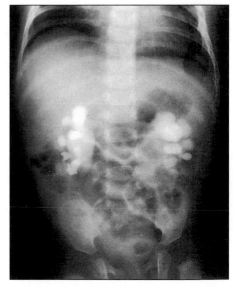

196

197

198

199

200

201

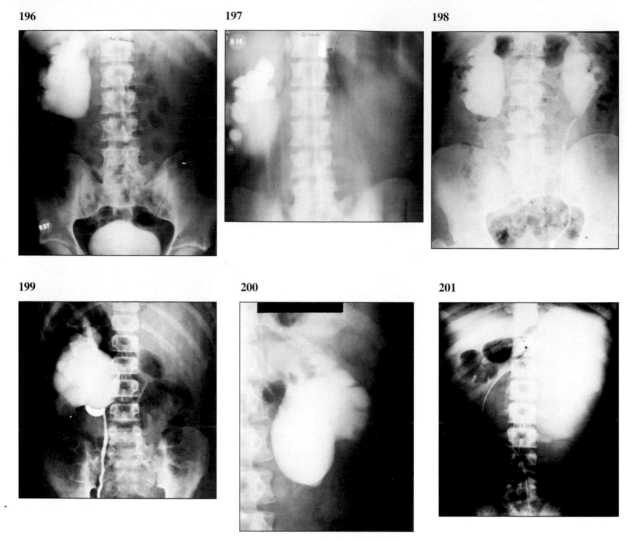

202

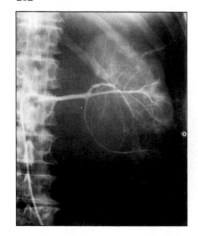

196 IVU of a hydronephrotic right kidney with no function on the left.

197 Tomogram revealing a large left renal outline.

198 Bilateral retrograde pyelogram confirming bilateral hydronephrosis.

199 PUJ obstruction due to a vessel crossing the ureter causing the pelvis to fall over the ureter, which then becomes acutely kinked, resulting in progressive hydronephrosis.

200 Considerable pelvic hydronephrosis with very early calyceal dilatation.

201 Gross hydronephrosis pushing the ureter across the midline.

202 Selective renal arteriogram showing a large dilated pelvis distorting the arterial system. The lower branch of the renal artery is coursing round the large hydronephrotic pelvis.

Renography in the diagnosis of PUJ obstruction

The main use of renography in PUJ obstruction is to differentiate between dilated obstruction and dilated nonobstructed collecting systems. The standard renogram curve in both situations is similar. However, if the urinary flow rate is increased by using frusemide the curves become dissimilar. In the dilated nonobstructed system, the diuresis induced by frusemide washes out the tracer, whereas diuresis in an obstructed system leads to retention of the tracer. In equivocal cases the frusemide may be given 15 minutes before the radiotracer. This ensures that the renogram is performed at the time of maximum diuresis.

203 Renogram of a patient with bilateral PUJ obstruction, showing retention of tracer despite administration of frusemide at 20 minutes.

— · — = Left renogram*
.... = Right renogram*
———— = Bladder activity
Urinary flow rate = 1.14ml/minute

Relative Function
Left = 50%
Right = 50%
Volume voided =40ml

204 IVU of a patient with bilateral hydronephrosis. A renogram is necessary to show whether obstruction is present.

205 Renogram of the same patient showing prompt washout of tracer on the left side before administration of frusemide, indicating a nonobstructed left kidney. On the right side, there is retention of tracer for up to 20 minutes, but following frusemide there is prompt washout, indicating a non-obstructed right kidney.

— · — = Left renogram*
.... = Right renogram*
———— = Bladder activity
Urinary flow rate = 14ml/minute

Relative Function
Left = 64%
Right = 36%
Volume voided =550ml

*The curves are not normalised and are background subtracted.

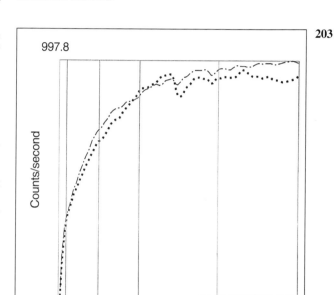

203

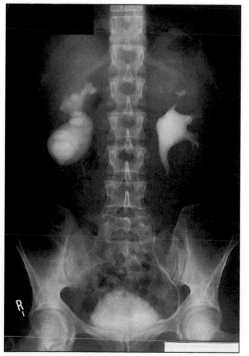

204

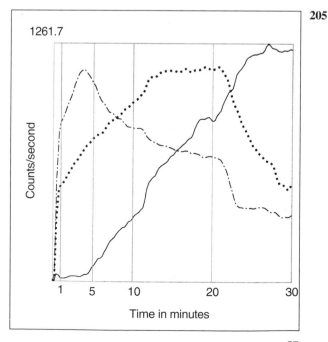

205

The Whitaker test

The Whitaker test (see Chapter 1, p. 27) can also be used to differentiate between an obstruction at the PUJ and a dilated nonobstructed renal pelvis.

206

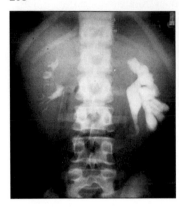

207

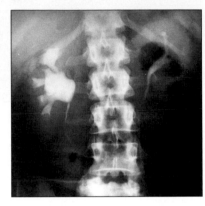

206 and 207 are two cases of hydro-nephrosis. The Whitaker test shows that **206** (tracing **208**) is obstructed and therefore requires surgery, while **207** is unobstructed (tracing **209**).

208

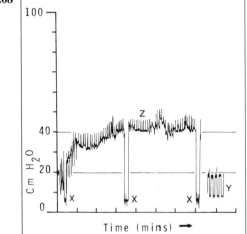

209

210

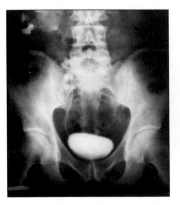

211

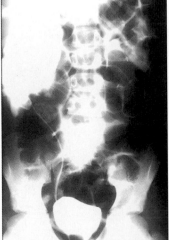

210 Complication of PUJ obstruction: infection. PUJ obstruction with a filling defect in the pelvis caused by mucopus. Obstruction can eventually lead to complete destruction of the kidney.

211 Complication of PUJ obstruction: rupture.

212, 213, 214 PUJ obstruction. Three pictures of the same hydro-nephrotic kidney. **212** shows the unopened specimen showing the dilation above the PUJ. **213** demonstrates the opened pelvis and ureter with no anatomical structural lesion at the PUJ. **214** is a close-up of the PUJ with the dilated pelvicalyceal system above.

212

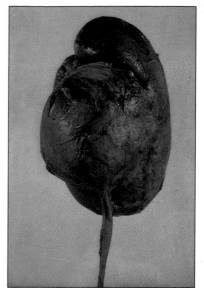

213

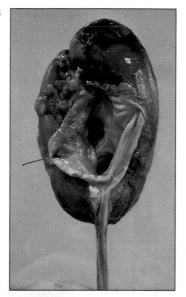

214

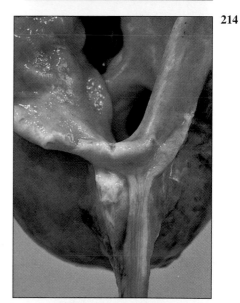

215

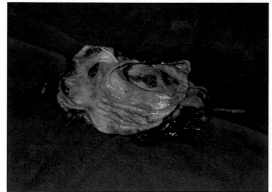

216

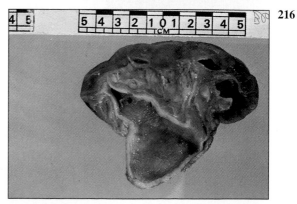

215 Typical longstanding obstruction, which has destroyed the renal parenchyma so that only a thin shell of renal tissue remains. Repeated attacks of infection lead to pyonephrosis which will rapidly destroy the kidney.

216 A kidney that has been completely destroyed by repeated infection.

Abnormalities of the ureter

217

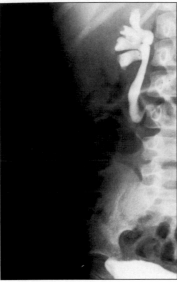

218

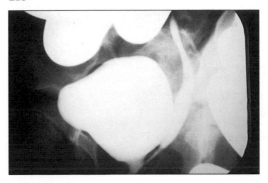

Vesicoureteric reflux may be congenital or acquired, and is covered in Chapter 3.

217 Retrocaval ureter in which the characteristic curve of the ureter is clearly seen. Retrocaval ureter is caused by persistence of the precursor of the inferior vena cava remaining anterior to the ureter.

218 Ectopic ureter. The ureter drains into the urethra below the bladder neck, causing continuous incontinence. It may also drain into the vagina.

Ureterocele

An ureterocele is a congenital cystic dilatation of the submucosal segment of the lower end of the ureter. It can be unilateral or bilateral, intravesical, or ectopic. An intravesical ureterocele may be associated with a single system, but may also be associated with the upper pole ureter of a duplex system (rarely the lower pole). In an ectopic ureterocele some portion of the ureterocele is permanently situated at the bladder neck or in the urethra, and the orifice may be in the bladder, bladder neck, or urethra.

219

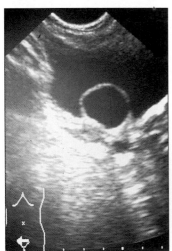

219 Ureterocele with calculus within. Note the acoustic shadow.

220

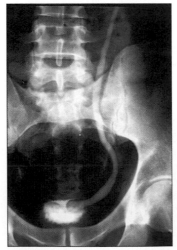

220 Unilateral ureterocele showing classical cobra head appearance.

221

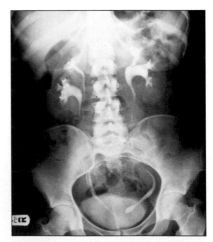

221 Bilateral ureterocele, the right being from the upper moiety of a duplex system.

222 Unilateral ureterocele affecting upper moiety of the duplex system with reflux into the lower moiety.

223 Ureteroceles can vary in size even in the same patient. This IVU shows a large right ureterocele and a small classical left cobra head ureterocele.

224 Prolapsing ureterocele is the commonest cause of retention in female infants.

225 Ureterocele showing a dilated thin mucosa.

226 Small ureterocele with a calculus *in situ*.

227, 228 KUB and IVU: stones can become quite large.

222

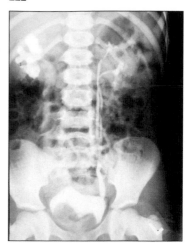

223

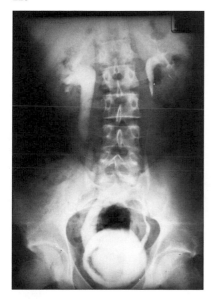

224

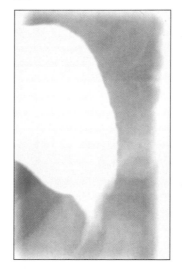

225

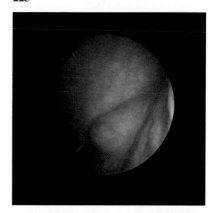

226

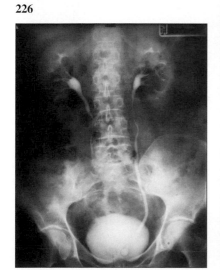

227

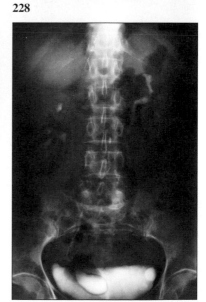

228

Megaureter

229

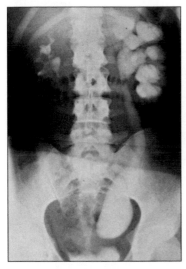

230

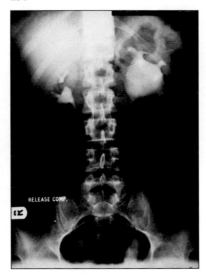

229 Megaureter is a ureter that is so dilated that effective peristalsis cannot occur. It may be primary, or secondary to bladder outflow obstruction. Primary megaureter can be obstructive or non-obstructive, refluxing or nonrefluxing, and unilateral or bilateral. Obstruction is due to a narrow segment at the lower end of the ureter.

230 Megaureter with PUJ obstruction.

Abnormalities of the urethra

Posterior urethral valves

Posterior urethral valves are the commonest cause of obstructive uropathy in boys and may be associated with bilateral hydronephrosis, which is detectable with antenatal ultrasound. Diagnosis is confirmed after birth by cystography.

231

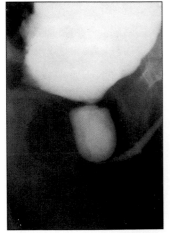

231 Micturating cystogram of infant with posterior urethral valves.

232

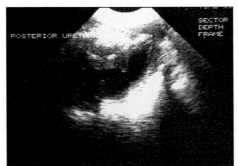

232 Ultrasound of posterior urethral valves shows a thick-walled bladder and a dilated posterior urethra.

233

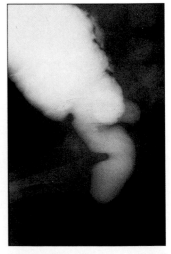

233 A more severe example of posterior urethral valves on cystography.

234 A specimen from a male infant who died 10 days after birth. Despite early detection of this condition by ultrasound some cases are too severe to benefit from treatment. Note the valves at the level of the verumontanum, the dilated posterior urethra, and the thick-walled bladder. There is also severe hydroureter and hydronephrosis with atrophy of the renal parenchyma.

235 IVU of an adolescent successfully treated for posterior urethral valves in childhood. Renal impairment continues throughout life and some survivors of this condition develop late-onset renal failure. The right kidney is nonfunctioning due to atrophy and the left kidney shows severe pelvicalyceal clubbing.

234

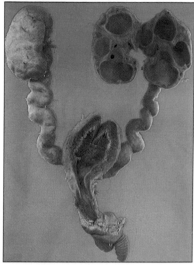

235

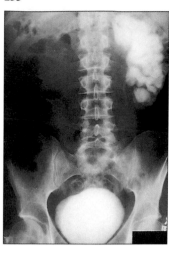

Prune belly syndrome

Prune belly syndrome is a rare syndrome of unknown aetiology. It occurs only in boys and involves absence of the abdominal wall muscles, gross dilatation of the urinary tract, and bilateral intra-abdominal testes. The kidneys are usually dysplastic, and the urinary tract is prone to infection, but long-term renal function is good in 50% of cases. Babies born with the prune belly syndrome are now becoming less common because it can be diagnosed as early as 15 weeks of gestation, at a time when a mother may choose termination of an affected fetus.

236

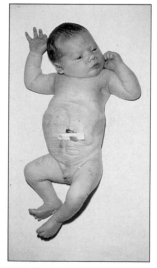

236 Boy with prune belly syndrome.

237

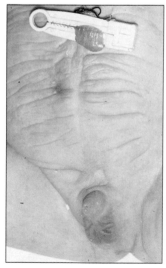

237 Close-up of abdomen shows prune-like appearance and empty scrotum.

238

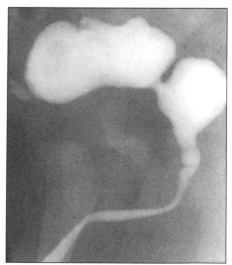

238 Cystogram of a boy with prune belly syndrome. There is often associated urethral irregularity, but rarely obstruction, and the bladder is characteristically hour-glass shaped, with a horizontal configuration, and a persistent urachal remnant, which may be patent.

239

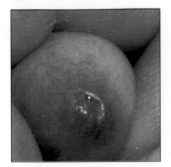

240

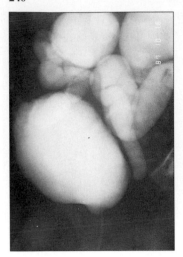

241

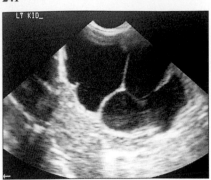

242

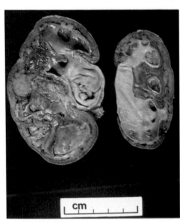

239 The urethra in the prune belly syndrome is occasionally atretic in which case the bladder empties via a persistent urachus or a vesicocutaneous fistula.

240 Cystogram of a boy with prune belly syndrome showing a large bladder with gross reflux into massively dilated ureters. Despite the alarming appearance renal function is often very good, but obstruction at any site in the urinary tract is difficult to diagnose with isotopic or pressure flow studies due to stasis in a high capacity, highly compliant system.

241 Ultrasound is useful for assessing the renal cortex, but cannot exclude obstruction. In this case gross dilatation of the collecting system with only a shell of renal cortex suggests atrophy.

242 Specimen from a 2-year-old boy with prune belly syndrome who died of septicaemia secoundary to infection in his dilated urinary tract. The kidney is full of pus and there is very little renal cortex.

Urethral duplication

Urethral duplication is very rare. The extra urethra may lie alongside the normal urethra, or may be dorsal or ventral.

243

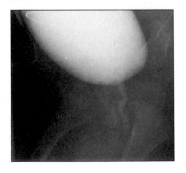

244

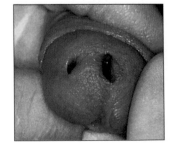

243 Micturating cystogram. In the Y-duplication shown here the second channel opens in the perineum, and the normal urethra is atretic.

244 Glans penis with two urethras side by side.

Exstrophy–epispadias complex

Abnormal development of the cloacal membrane during the first four weeks of embryonic life results in a spectrum of anomalies ranging from the lesser abnormality of epispadias without exstrophy, through classical bladder exstrophy and its variants, to the very severe disorder of cloacal exstrophy (not shown).

245

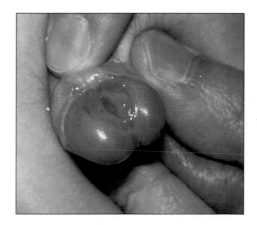

246

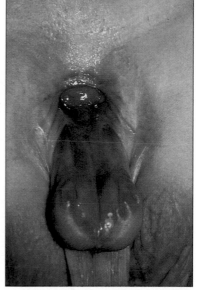

245 Glandular epispadias. Complete epispadias without exstrophy occurs in 1 in 200,000 males and 1 in 400,000 females. In glandular epispadias the patient is usually continent, and the glans is flattened with a dorsal split.

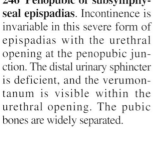

246 Penopubic or subsymphyseal epispadias. Incontinence is invariable in this severe form of epispadias with the urethral opening at the penopubic junction. The distal urinary sphincter is deficient, and the verumontanum is visible within the urethral opening. The pubic bones are widely separated.

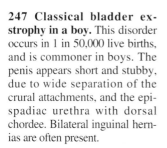

247

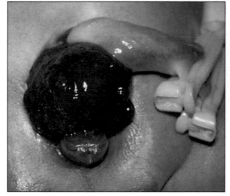

248

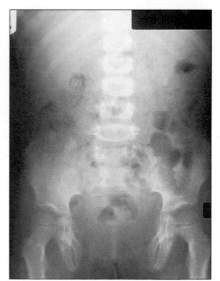

247 Classical bladder exstrophy in a boy. This disorder occurs in 1 in 50,000 live births, and is commoner in boys. The penis appears short and stubby, due to wide separation of the crural attachments, and the epispadiac urethra with dorsal chordee. Bilateral inguinal hernias are often present.

248 Plain abdominal radiograph of a girl with bladder exstrophy. The condition is associated with rotational deformity of the pelvic girdle, resulting in wide separation of the pubic bones, which are held together by a symphyseal band.

Hypospadias

The hypospadiac anomaly (which is very common) occurs later in embryonic development than the exstrophy–epispadias complex, and is probably due to relative androgen insensitivity of the genital tubercle after the sixth week of gestation. Hypospadias is classified according to the position of the meatus, which is glandular or coronal in 70% of cases. There is usually an associated ventral chordee, which is worse when the meatus is more proximal.

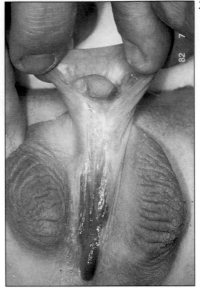

249

249 Severe hypospadias. A proximal hypospadiac meatus is rare, and in this case is associated with a bifid scrotum. Although the perineal and scrotal varieties of hypospadias may occur in intersex states, the majority of cases of hypospadias are minor, and not associated with ambiguous genitalia.

3 Inflammatory diseases of the urinary tract

Pyelonephritis

Acute bacterial pyelonephritis is usually a dramatic febrile illness presenting with loin pain and rigors. Chronic bacterial pyelonephritis is insidious and may lead to hypertension and renal failure: it rarely occurs unless an abnormality exists somewhere in the outflow tract.

Bacteria may reach the kidney by the blood stream, lymph or via the ureter, but it is likely that most infections are ascending infections. The bacteria involved are usually Gram-negative bacilli, particularly *Escherichia coli* and *Bacillus proteus*, but may also be Gram-positive organisms including *Streptococcus faecalis* and *Staphylococcus albus*. These organisms can produce inflammatory disorders at all levels of the urinary tract.

Chronic pyelonephritis has been overdiagnosed because of the assumption that all coarsely scarred kidneys result from urinary tract infection. This is not so; similar changes can result from vascular abnormalities, analgesic abuse, or irradiation. In the absence of obstruction or proof of infection, it is better to use the term interstitial nephritis for such kidneys.

This chapter also covers parasitic infestations such as chyluria (bilharzia merits a chapter of its own, see Chapter 5), and the inflammatory conditions produced by specific disease such as diabetes and analgesic abuse. The rarer conditions of obscure aetiology such as interstitial cystitis, retroperitoneal fibrosis, and malakoplakia are also presented.

250

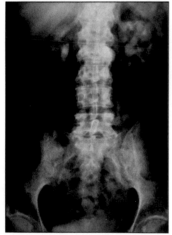

250 IVU showing severe bilateral pyelonephritis with reduction in kidney size, cortical scarring, and calyceal dilatation and deformity.

251

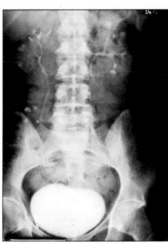

251 IVU showing less marked bilateral changes.

252

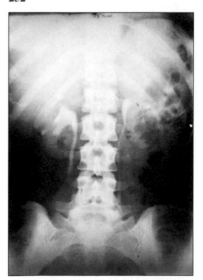

252 Changes may be much less severe and a scar with a related superficial calyx in the right kidney indicates focal damage.

253

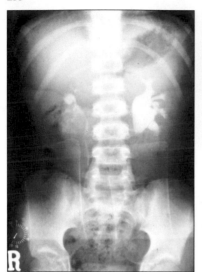

254

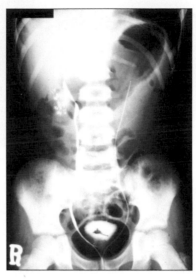

253, 254 When there is only minimal function in the IVU (here on the right side) retrograde pyelography will delineate the small, severely damaged kidney.

255

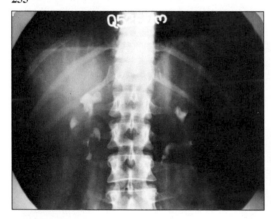

256

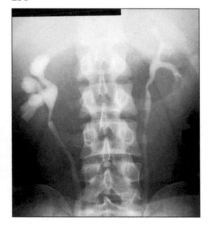

255 Changes may be confined to one pole and are often seen affecting the upper pole, as in this IVU.

256 Calyceal clubbing is well demonstrated here.

257

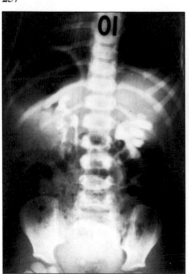

258

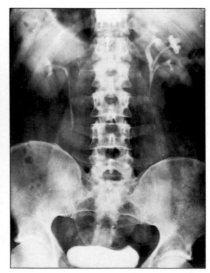

257 Calyceal clubbing. The severity of the process often varies between the two kidneys.

258 Calyceal clubbing. Sometimes the disease process is effectively unilateral.

Vesicoureteric reflux

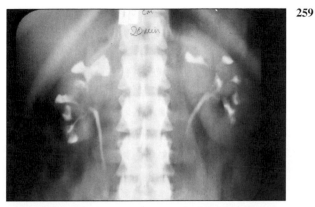

259

259 Pyelonephritis in children and adolescent females gives rise to the suspicion of primary vesicoureteric reflux. This IVU shows classical cortical thinning and calyceal damage in a 19-year-old girl with a 10-year history of urinary tract infections.

Micturating cystourethrogram

The micturating cystourethrogram (MCU) is an essential investigation in all patients with recurrent urinary tract infection. Reflux is recorded in 5 grades. Ultrasound and radionuclide studies can also be used.

260

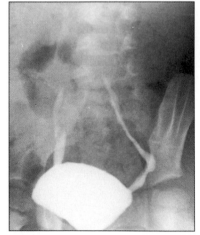

260 Grade I reflux.

261

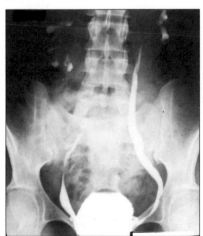

261 Grade II reflux.

262

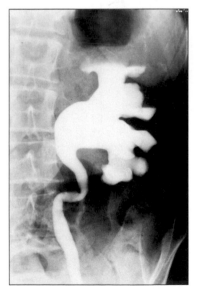

262 Grade III reflux.

263

264

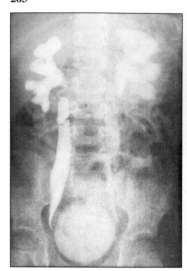

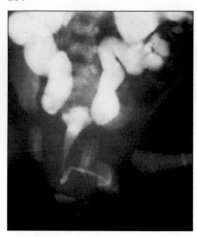

263 Grade IV reflux.

264 Grade V reflux.

265

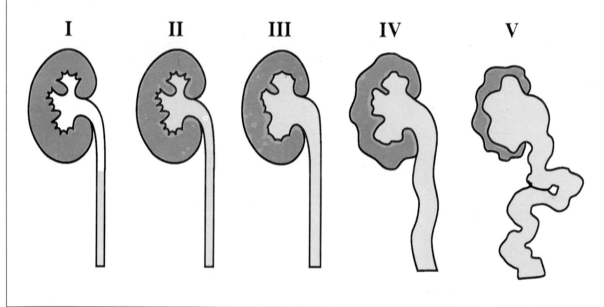

265 Grade of vesicoureteric reflux. International classification.

Comparative classifications					
International	I	II	III	IV	V
Dwoskin and Perlmutter	IIA	IIB	III	III	IV
Winberg *et al.*	I	II	II	III	IV
Rolleston *et al.*	I	I	II	III	III
Smellie *et al.**	I	II/III	II/III	IV	IV

*Smellie *et al.*, classification: grade II is 'filling reflux' only when voiding; grade III is reflux when voiding or at rest.

266 Bilateral reflux may not cause severe renal changes, as in this MCU of a young male.

267 Filling reflux. During the filling phase of the MCU Grade I low pressure reflux is seen on the right.

266

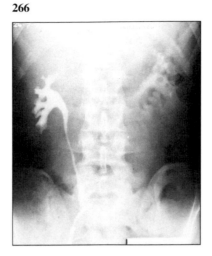

267

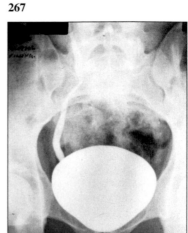

268 Voiding reflux. Bilateral high pressure reflux occurs on voiding.

269 Grade IV reflux. Full length film of gross voiding reflux with marked cortical thinning.

Congenital anatomical ureteric anomalies may also give rise to reflux. This young woman had a complete right duplex ureteric system (**270, 271**).

270 IVU showing right duplex system with ureterocele and normal left system.

271 MCU. Reflux is seen into the lower moiety of the right kidney with that ureter entering the bladder above the upper moiety ureter. This second ureter terminated in a small ureterocele with obstruction. No reflux or obstruction occurred on the left side.

268

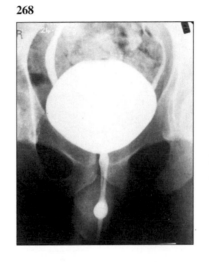

269

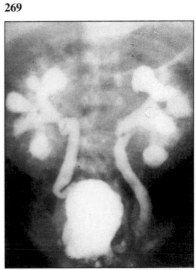

270

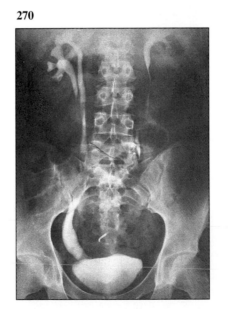

271

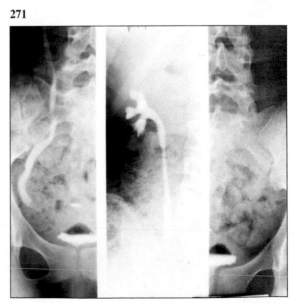

272

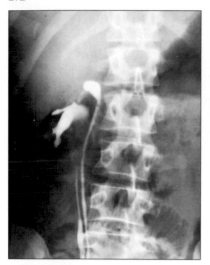

273

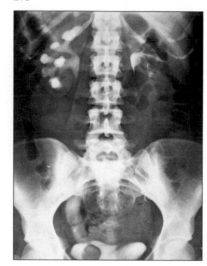

274

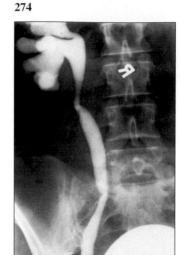

272 Reflux may occur in both ureters of a duplex system.

273, 274 Reflux may also be secondary to iatrogenic damage to the ureteric orifices in endoscopic procedures and here followed endoscopic incision of a uretero-cele. **273** IVU showing right ureterocele; **274** MCU after endoscopic incision.

275

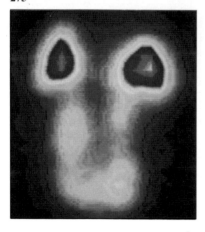

276

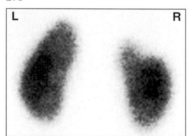

277

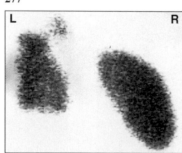

Radionuclide DMSA scanning

Radionuclide DMSA scanning is useful in evaluation of reflux and in the demonstration of scars and thinning of the cortex using the DMSA technique.

275 Isotope cystogram showing bilateral reflux.

276 Right upper polar scar only, but with diminuition of function to 45% on that side.

277 DMSA scan showing gross scarring and reduction in size of left kidney.

278

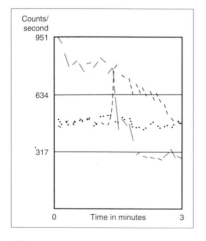

Voiding radionuclide cystogram

This technique is also useful in the evaluation of reflux in these patients.

278 Voiding study demonstrating left-sided grade III reflux.
－－－－－ = Left renogram*
• • • • • = Right renogram*
.... = Bladder activity
  *The curves are not normalised and are background subtracted.

279

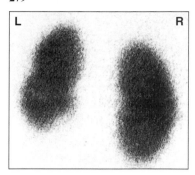

279 Mid pole scar demonstrated by DMSA scanning in patient studied in **278**. Left mid pole scars with nearly 10% reduction in function on that side.

280

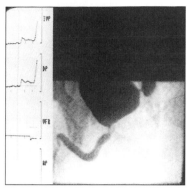

280 Video urodynamic study showing intravesical pressure, detrusor pressure, flow rate, and intra-abdominal (rectal) pressure with video image in a boy with bladder neck obstruction and reflux.

281

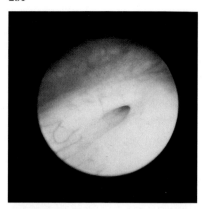

281 Refluxing ureteric orifice, which is gaping, hooded, and pale. The contraction of this type of orifice is usually weak.

Reflux can also be associated with obstruction.

282

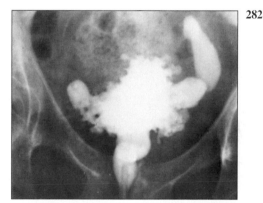

282 Reflux may also result from obstruction to the lower tract or a neuropathic bladder disorder, as seen here.

Pathological changes in pyelonephritis

283

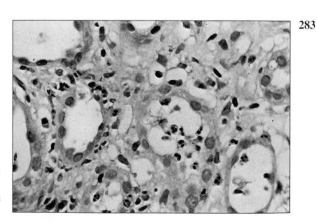

283 Acute pyelonephritis. Section from a patient with proven urinary tract infection, showing neutrophil polymorphonuclear leucocyte infiltration of the tubular epithelium and lumen. *(H&E × 256)*

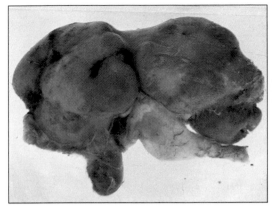

284 Chronic pyelonephritis. Outer surface of a coarsely scarred kidney (formalin fixed).

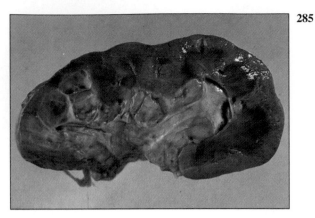

285 Chronic pyelonephritis. Cut surface of a coarsely scarred kidney showing distortion of the pelvicalyceal system and loss of renal parenchyma in the scarred areas.

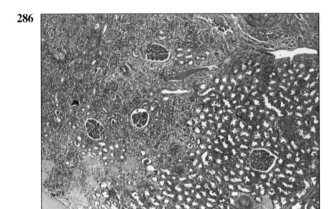

286 Chronic pyelonephritis. Section showing an area of relatively normal parenchyma (on the right hand side of the field) with a very abnormal one (on the left). In the abnormal area the striking feature is the tubular damage and inflammatory cell infiltrate in the interstitium. There are three relatively well-preserved glomeruli present in the middle of this area, but some sclerotic ones are present in the bottom left hand corner. This patchy involvement is a feature of chronic pyelonephritis. *(H&E × 26)*

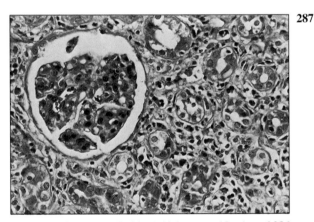

287 Chronic pyelonephritis. A higher magnification of **286** showing chronic inflammatory cell infiltration in the interstitium with a preserved glomerulus. *(H&E × 160)*

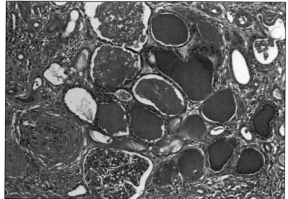

288 Chronic pyelonephritis. Marked tubular dilatation, the lumina being filled with eosinophilic protein casts. This appearance is similar to the colloid-filled follicles in the thyroid and is often called thyroidisation. *(H&E × 64)*

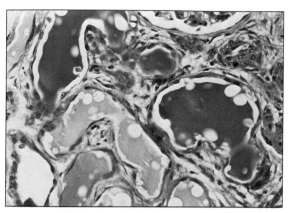

289 Chronic pyelonephritis. Higher magnification of tubules similar to those in **288**, showing the marked flattening of the tubular epithelium. *(H&E × 160)*

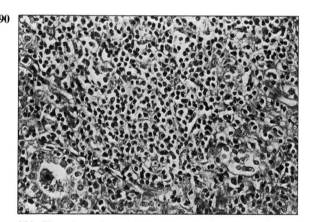

290 Chronic pyelonephritis. A section of medulla showing marked infiltration of the interstitium with inflammatory cells, with some entering the tubules. *(H&E × 160)*

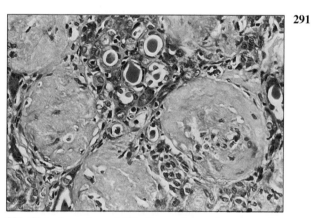

291 Chronic pyelonephritis. In an advanced stage scarring and hyalinisation may predominate over inflammatory cell infiltration. This section shows hyalinised glomeruli and some protein casts in atrophic tubules. *(H&E × 160)*

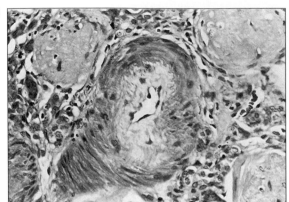

292 Chronic pyelonephritis. Arterial changes are often prominent, especially in advanced disease. This section shows an artery with marked intimal proliferation in the middle of the field. Some hyalinised glomeruli are present. In advanced disease it may be difficult to decide whether the process is infective in origin. *(H&E × 160)*

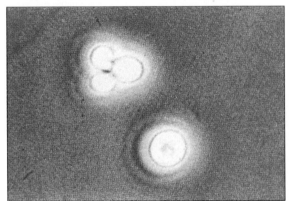

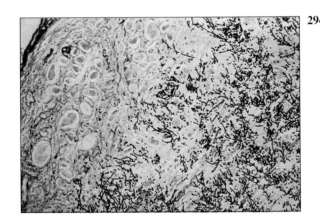

293, 294 Fungal infections may also cause renal inflammatory disease as in candidiasis of the kidney. Renal candidiasis presenting as a *Candida* ball usually results from a widespread overwhelming fungal infection in the seriously debilitated patient. **293** shows budding forms of *Candida albicans*. **294** is a silver preparation showing fungal hyphae (black) growing in tissue.

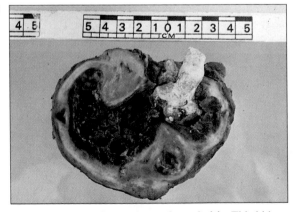

295 Xanthogranulomatous pyelonephritis. This kidney contains a staghorn calculus. The pelvis is dilated and haemorrhagic. The renal parenchyma is scarred and contains yellow-orange areas. Histology of these areas shows many lipid-laden histiocytes with multinucleate giant cells, the pattern of xanthogranulomatous pyelonephritis.

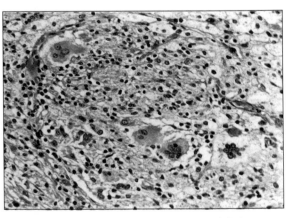

296 Xanthogranulomatous pyelonephritis is a term applied to a form of chronic pyelonephritis in which a heavy infiltrate of histiocytes (macrophages) is prominent among the chronic inflammatory cells. These cells have foamy cytoplasm caused by their lipid content, and some are multinucleate. The appearances are similar to those seen in xanthoma, which usually lacks other inflammatory cells. *(H&E × 80)*

297

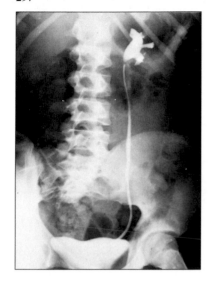

298

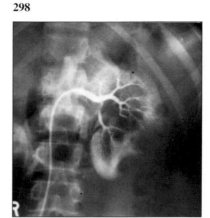

299

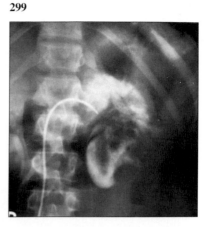

297 Abscess formation may occur in distinct areas of the renal cortex producing a renal carbuncle, which is usually staphylococcal in origin, but may be secondary to suppurative pyelonephritis. Notoriously difficult to diagnose, the patients are ill, febrile, and often develop flank pain late. The urine may be sterile. Pyelography and retrograde studies may be unhelpful, although pelvicalyceal distortion may occur and the renal outline may be altered.

298, 299 Arteriography demonstrates an irregular loss of renal tissue at the lower pole.

Perinephric abscess

Perinephric abscesses almost always arise from the kidney, most frequently in association with stone disease. The abscess lies around the kidney, usually confined by Gerota's fascia, and may point through the skin or drain into the colon. Occasionally it may track below the inguinal ligament or up to the diaphragm.

300

300 A gas-filled abscess cavity.

301 Retrograde study shows compression and medial deviation of the pelvicalyceal system.

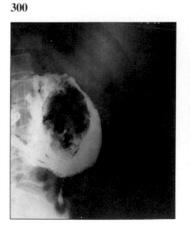

301

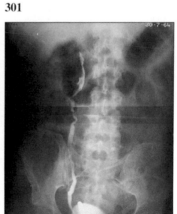

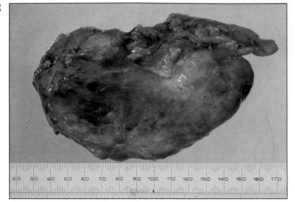

302

302 Pyonephrotic kidney: outer surface. Pyonephrosis is usually a result of infection by pyogenic organisms after obstruction by a stone or of a hydronephrotic kidney with pelviureteric obstruction. This leads to rapid destruction of the kidney.

303 Pyonephrosis. The cut surface of the specimen shown in **302**. The dilated pelvis was filled with pus and abscesses are present in the renal parenchyma and communicate with the pelvis.

304 Pyonephrosis. Section from near the pelvis. It shows many neutrophil polymorphonuclear leucocytes and some larger cells with foamy cytoplasm (histiocytes with ingested material). *(H&E × 256)*

303

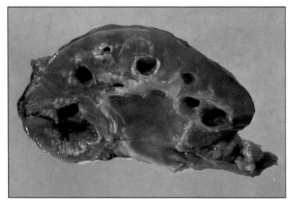

304

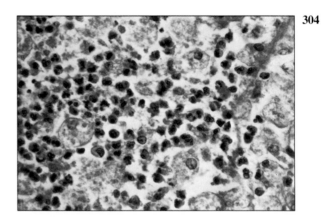

305

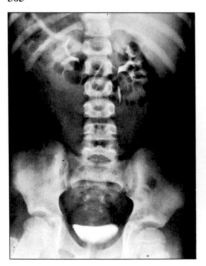

306

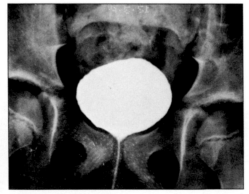

307

305, 306, 307, Localisation studies for bacterial infection are valuable in the assessment of recurrent or chronic urinary tract infections. This child with recurrent urinary tract infection had a normal IVU (**305**), no reflux on the MCU (**306**), and localisation showed infection confined to the bladder alone (**307**). Upper tract localisation (UTL) is an investigation that is now only occasionally warranted, but it remains a valuable adjunct to the management of urinary tract infection. Under a diuresis, cystoscopic specimens are collected from the bladder and both ureters.

UTL F 8 years: Bladder infection

Specimen	*Bacterial count/ml*
CU	*Proteus mirabilis* 10^6
WB	*Proteus mirabilis* 60 cols
RK1–5	No growth
LK1–5	No growth

CU = cystopic urine specimen.
WB = washed bladder specimen.
RK/LK1–5 = 5 consecutive ureteric specimens of urine
from each kidney.

308 Upper tract infections may be unilateral or bilateral
and are frequently associated with stone disease. Left-sided
infection is confirmed here in a hypoplastic kidney.

308

**UTL F 53 years: Left renal infection,
hypoplastic kidney**

Specimen	Bacterial count/ml
CU	Escherichia coli 10^6
WB	Escherichia coli 20 cols
RK1–5	No growth
LK1	Escherichia coli 10^4
LK2–5	Escherichia coli 10^6

309

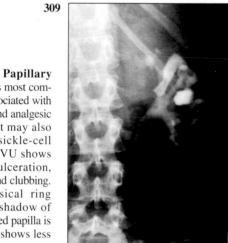

**309, 310 Papillary
necrosis** is most com-
monly associated with
diabetes and analgesic
abuse, but may also
occur in sickle-cell
disease. IVU shows
calyceal ulceration,
scarring and clubbing.
The classical ring
negative shadow of
the sloughed papilla is
seen. **310** shows less
marked changes.

310

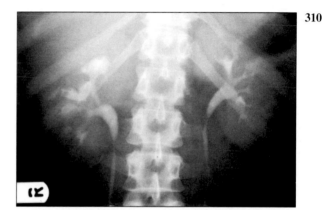

311

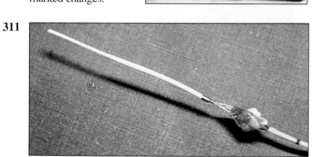

312

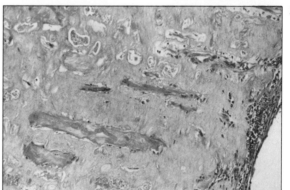

313

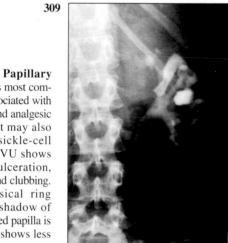

311 The sloughed papilla causing ureteric obstruction,
extracted endoscopically with the dormia basket.

312 Papillary necrosis. Section showing the structured
necrosis seen in papillary necrosis. Note the ghost outlines of
the structure of the papilla with virtual absence of nuclear
staining. *(H&E × 26)*

313 Papillary necrosis. Postmortem specimen of a kidney
from a diabetic patient. The extreme pallor of the papillae is
caused by necrosis (formalin fixed).

Complications of diabetes

314

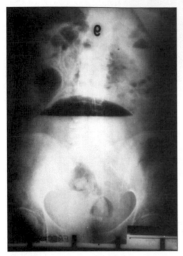

315

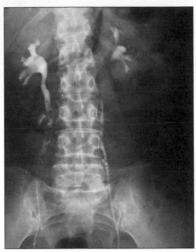

316

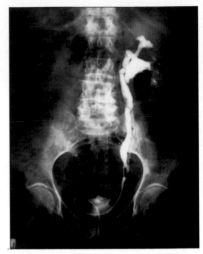

314 Infection with gas-forming organisms may occur in diabetes, giving rise to gas in the bladder, and here in the right kidney as well.

315 Chronic bacterial infection may give rise to the pyelographic changes of pyelo-ureteritis cystica.

316 These changes may progress to marked ureteric changes with irregularity and filling defects shown on the ascending study. The histological appearances are the same as those of cystitis cystica.

Pelvic lipomatosis
Pelvic lipomatosis is a condition of unknown origin in which the pelvis is filled by lipomatous tissue.

317

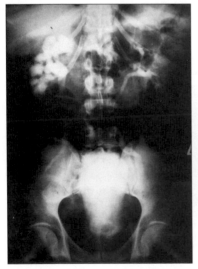

318

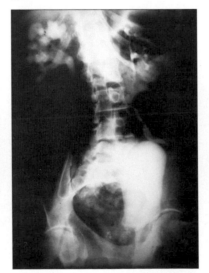

319

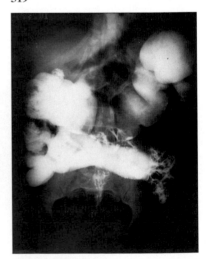

317 Bladder elevated and right ureter obstructed causing early hydronephrosis. Note the dark shadow in the pelvis.

318 Oblique view of the same patient.

319 Barium enema to show the rectal string sign caused by external pressure of the lipomatous tissue (dark shadow) on the rectum.

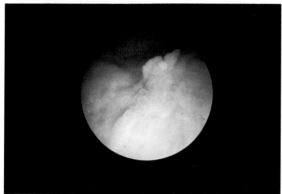

320 Intra-abdominal chronic inflammatory disease such as diverticulitis or Crohn's disease may lead to fistulation to the ureter or bladder. The characteristic granulations are seen around the fistulous opening at endoscopy.

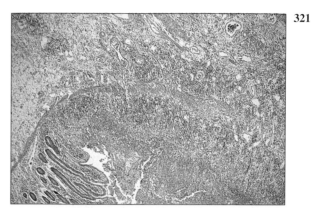

321 Crohn's disease is a chronic inflammatory disease of the alimentary tract, particularly affecting the terminal ileum. The cause is unknown. The inflammation spreads through the wall of the bowel and may penetrate other organs, including the bladder. This picture shows an ulcerated piece of small bowel mucosa with inflammation spreading into the wall. *(H&E)*

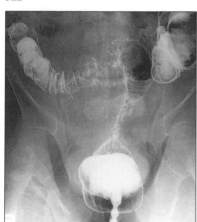
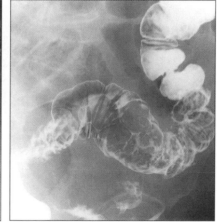

322 Vesicocolic fistula. Vesical shadow seen superimposed on the rectum as a result of contrast medium reaching the bladder via the fistula.

323 Fistula demonstrated.

Idiopathic retroperitoneal fibrosis

Idiopathic retroperitoneal fibrosis (RPF), first described by Ormand in 1948, is a proliferation of fibrous tissue, often with blood vessels and other inflammatory cells. It develops in the retroperitoneum, usually centred around the aorta, often low down extending upwards, and tends to involve the ureters, causing hydronephrosis and resulting in renal failure. Similar cases were associated with methysergide therapy for migraine. It is important to remember that some neoplasms in the retroperitoneum can stimulate a fibroblastic response, which can be mistaken for idiopathic RPF. There is also a possibility that this condition arises in association with beta-blockade therapy, and it also occurs in relation to inflammatory aneurysms of the abdominal aorta. In some cases, problems with diagnosis may arise since calcification can occur in plaques of RPF.

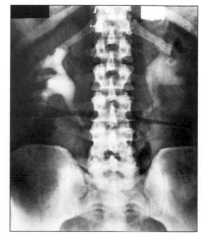

324 Bilateral hydronephrosis typical of RPF is seen in this IVU.

325

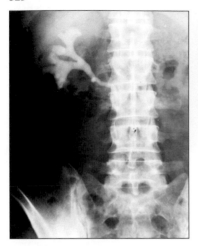

326

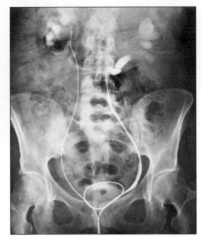

325 Gross medial indrawing of the ureter is present in this patient whose left kidney was removed earlier for 'hydronephrosis of unknown cause'.

326 Bilateral ureteric catheterisation shows the indrawn ureters, but catheters may pass without any difficulty.

327

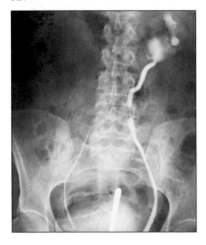

328

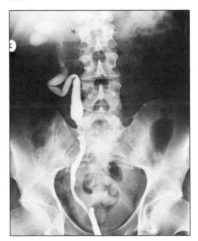

327, 328 Ascending ureterography using the bulb-ended ureteric catheter is diagnostic in that the extrinsic compression of the ureter by fibrosis is delineated.

329

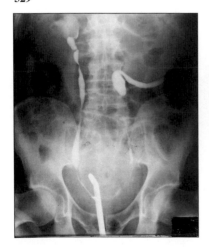

330

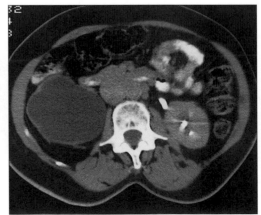

329 A long ureteric stricture may also be found.

330 CT scan showing a normal left kidney and a grossly hydronephrotic right kidney where the ureter has been blocked by involvement in an aortic aneurysm. Para-aortic inflammatory tissue extends round the aorta and inferior vena cava and draws in both ureters.

331

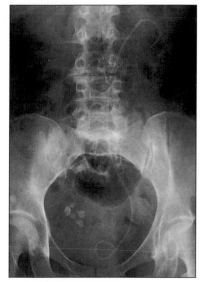

332

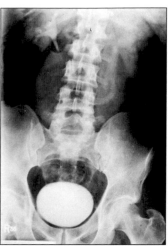

333

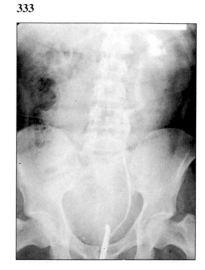

334

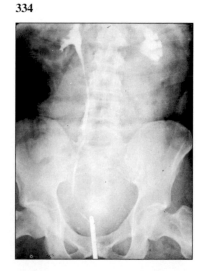

331 A double pigtail stent placed in the left ureter demonstrates the medial deviation of the ureter that is characteristic of this condition.

332, 333, 334 The condition usually affects both ureters, but it can present with uni-lateral obstruction. The IVU and left ascending ureterogram demonstrate RPF affecting the left ureter while the right ureterogram is normal. Exploration and biopsy confirmed the diagnosis.

335

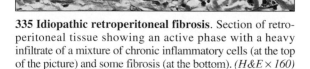

335 Idiopathic retroperitoneal fibrosis. Section of retro-peritoneal tissue showing an active phase with a heavy infiltrate of a mixture of chronic inflammatory cells (at the top of the picture) and some fibrosis (at the bottom). *(H&E × 160)*

336

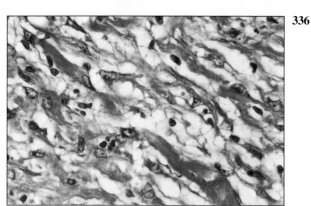

336 Idiopathic retroperitoneal fibrosis. Section showing more mature dense fibrous tissue with little inflammatory cell infiltrate. *(H&E × 256)*

Cystitis

337

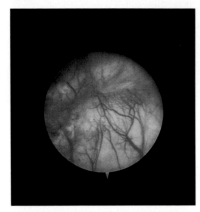

337 Endoscopic changes in the bladder show the injected appearance of slightly engorged mucosal blood vessels in the early stages.

338

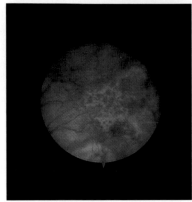

338 A patchy inflammation will be seen with mild cystitis.

339

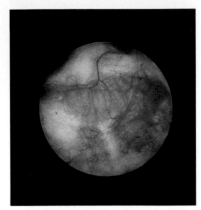

339 A more severe form.

340

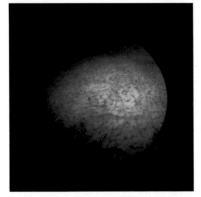

340 Punctate haemorrhages are noted.

341

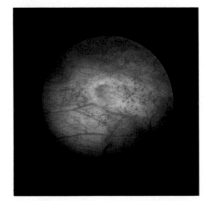

341 Inflammation around a ureteric orifice.

342

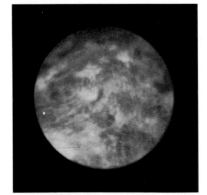

342 Florid acute cystitis.

343

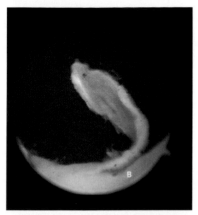

343 Cystourethritis may be accompanied by inflammatory polypi at the bladder neck. There is a variable degree of bladder neck inflammation.

344

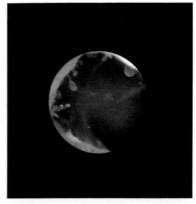

344 The rarer polypi at the male bladder neck.

345

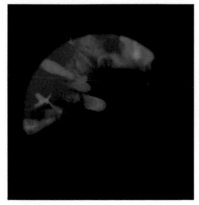

345 Florid posterior urethritis with polypi.

346

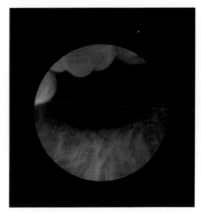

346 Prostatitis gives rise to this characteristic appearance of an intensely red and oedematous bladder neck and prostatic urethral mucosa.

347

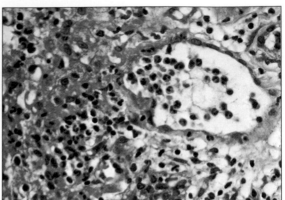

348

347 Acute cystitis. An oedematous mucosa with very congested blood vessels. Red cells spill out of the vessels where margination of neutrophil polymorphonuclear leucocytes is seen. This is basically an early vascular phase of the acute inflammatory reaction. Later in the process one of the elements of the reaction may predominate, giving a picture that may be described as bullous, fibrinous, purulent, or haemorrhagic. *(H&E × 256)*

348 Acute cystitis. A severe acute inflammatory reaction. This is cystitis induced by cyclophosphamide therapy. It becomes chronic and results in a small contracted bladder. *(H&E × 256)*

349

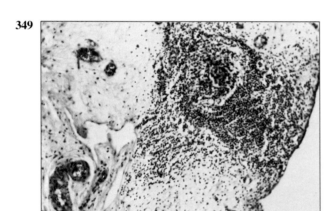

350

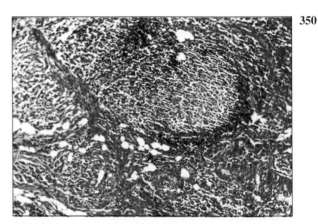

349 Chronic cystitis. An attenuated epithelium covering thickened connective tissue in which there is a heavy, but patchy, infiltrate of chronic inflammatory cells, mainly lymphocytes. *(H&E × 64)*

350 Chronic cystitis. Wall of the bladder with a heavy lymphoid infiltrate in which the aggregates of lymphoid cells have germinal centres. This pattern is often called follicular cystitis. *(H&E × 160)*

351

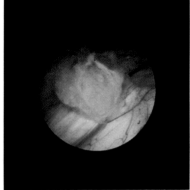

352

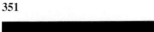

353

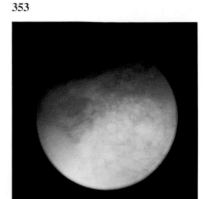

351 Fibromucous plaques. With more longlasting infection fibromucous plaques may be deposited on the urothelial surface.

352 Bladder bullae may also be noted. This process is entirely benign. Inflammatory proliferative conditions are also found in the bladder and include cystitis cystica and glandularis.

353 Cystitis cystica with clear cysts raised above the mucosa.

354

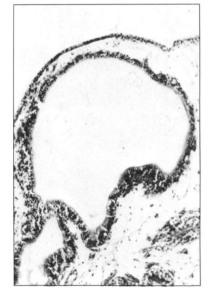

355

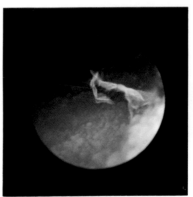

356

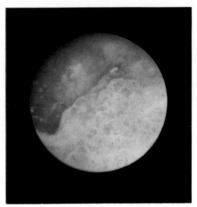

355, 356 Cystitis glandularis shows more florid cystic changes, and the bladder may show a 'cobble-stone' appearance.

354 Cystitis cystica. Attenuated epithelium (at the top) is spread out over a cystically dilated cavity lined with transitional epithelium. There are a few chronic inflammatory cells in the connective tissue (see also **512**, p. 120). *(H&E×64)*

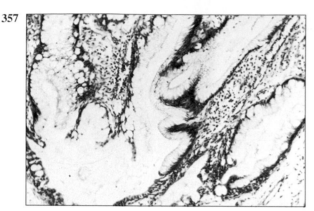

357 Cystitis glandularis. In the wall of the bladder there are cystic spaces lined mainly by tall columnar epithelium, which distinguishes this condition from cystitis cystica. *(H&E × 64)*

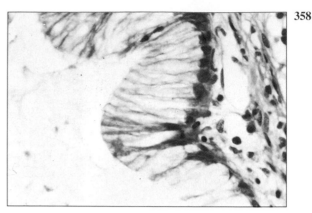

358 Cystitis glandularis. A higher magnification of ×85 showing the columnar epithelium, which is very different from the normal transitional epithelium. Adenocarcinoma may sometimes arise in this type of epithelium. *(H&E × 256)*

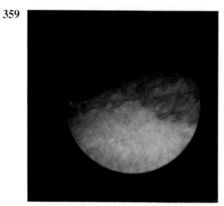

359 Squamous metaplasia of the trigone. The well-demarcated white edge of squamous metaplasia of the trigone is entirely benign, presents itself in women, and probably has hormonal causes.

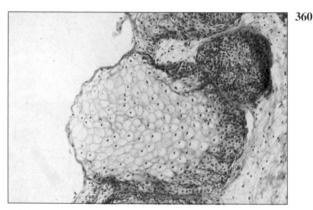

360 Squamous metaplasia of the trigone. Bladder biopsy from the trigone, where the normal transitional epithelium shows a squamoid maturation towards the surface, although it is not keratinising. *(H&E × 64)*

361 **362**

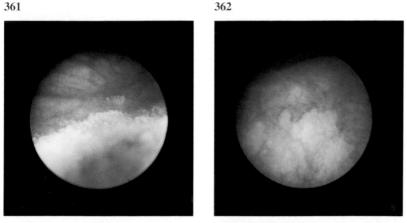

363

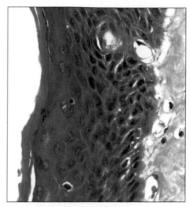

361, 362 Another form of squamous metaplasia occurs with chronic irritation of the bladder and this more widespread form, which is shown, is often called leukoplakia. It is of more sinister significance because neoplasms can develop in such areas.

363 Leukoplakia. Section of bladder mucosa showing squamous epithelium that is keratinising. The epithelial cells show mild atypia and the underlying connective tissue shows some hyalinisation. Moist keratin appears as a white plaque on visual examination. Not all keratinising areas on mucosal surfaces are premalignant. *(H&E × 256)*

364

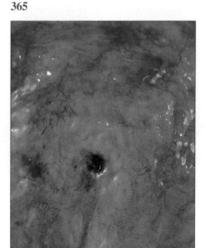

365

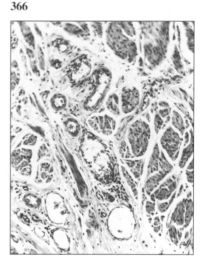

366

364 Interstitial cystitis, originally described in women by Hunner in 1915, is a chronic and painful irritable bladder syndrome, of unknown origin. The endoscopic appearance is characteristic with the radiate flare haemorrhages and ulcers in the bladder dome. Despite the sometimes localised ulcers, the changes are widespread in the bladder wall. The bladder may become progressively smaller and fibrotic.

365 Hunner's ulcer. Postmortem specimen of opened bladder showing the classical red mucosal flares surrounding an ulcerated area.

366 Hunner's ulcer. Fibrosis and chronic inflammatory cells extend down into the muscle. *(H&E × 64)*

367

368

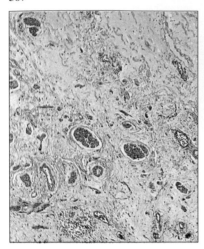

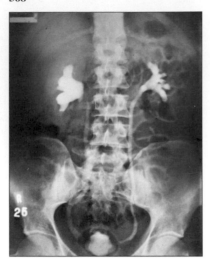

367 Hunner's ulcer. This section, in which fibrous tissue is stained green, shows the fibrosis in the wall, which leads to a small contracted bladder. *(Trichrome × 64)*

368 Eosinophilic cystitis. This is a rare form of inflammatory interstitial bladder disease and is characterised by gross frequency, usually in men. The IVU shows the thickened bladder with compression of the intramural ureters leading to obstruction of the upper tracts. Tuberculosis must always be excluded.

369

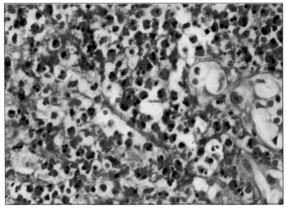

370

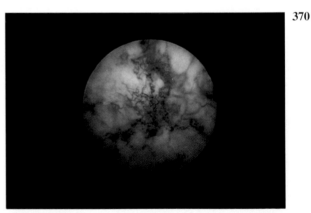

369 Eosinophilic cystitis. Section of the bladder showing a heavy infiltration of inflammatory cells in which the predominant cell is the eosinophil with a bilobed nucleus and bright eosinophilic, granular cytoplasm. *(H&E × 256)*

370 Irradiation cystitis is included as a form of 'inflammatory' cystitis. The endoscopic appearance is that of prominent vessels and blotchy haemorrhages interspersed with white atrophic areas of mucosa. This bleeds easily with bladder distension.

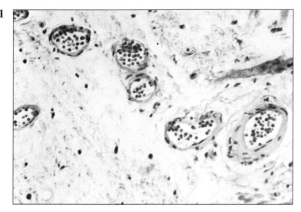

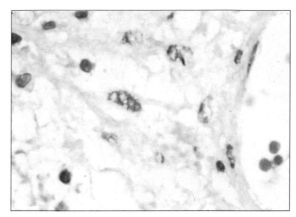

371 Irradiation cystitis. Telangiectatic blood vessels are prominent in this section of a post-irradiation bladder. *(H&E × 80)*

372 Irradiation cystitis. Fibrosis occurs in the wall of irradiated bladders and the fibroblasts often have an abnormal appearance. In this section the nuclei of fibroblasts are vacuolated; this is a characteristic post-irradiation appearance. *(H&E × 256)*

Malakoplakia

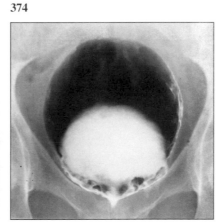

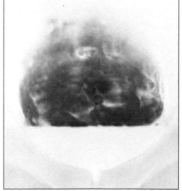

374, 375 Double contrast cystography shows the vesical plaques of malakoplakia.

373 Malakoplakia. This rare granulomatous lesion is almost totally confined to the urinary tract and was first described by Michaelis and Gutmann in 1902. Occurring predominantly in women, it is probably a reaction to *Escherichia coli* and usually presents with chronic cystitis, but can affect the upper tracts. In this IVU there is minimal function on the right side and obstruction to the left ureter.

376   **377**   **378**

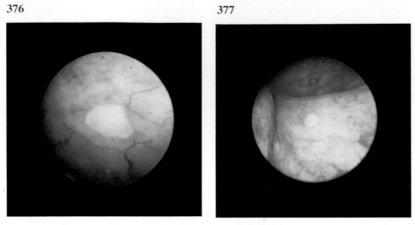

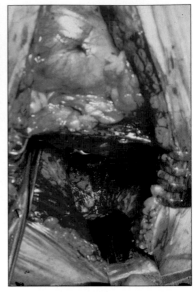

376, 377   **Endoscopic appearance of the soft, yellow plaques**.

378 Surgical appearance. Plaques can also be observed at open cystotomy.

379   **380**

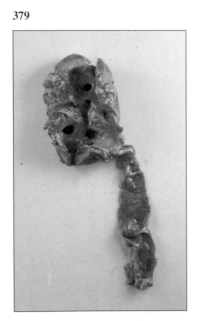

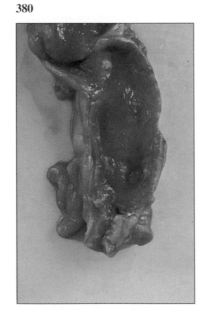

379, 380 Nephroureterectomy specimen showing gross hydronephrosis and hydroureter due to the stricture of the lower ureter caused by malakoplakia.

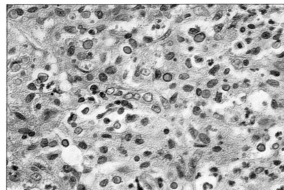

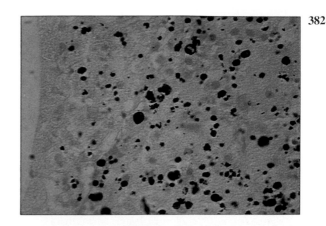

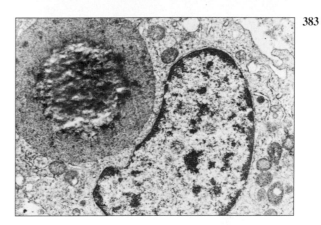

381 Malakoplakia. Sheets of histiocytes and some neutrophilic polymorphonuclear leucocytes. In the histiocytes some of the blue staining bodies are nuclei (with a vesicular predominantly oval appearance), but others appear as rather empty blue bodies, some laminated. These are Michaelis–Gutmann bodies. *(H&E × 256)*

382 Malakoplakia. This stain shows the calcium (black) present in Michaelis–Gutmann bodies. *(Von Kossa × 256)*

383 Michaelis–Gutmann body. An electron micrograph of a histiocyte showing its nucleus (more or less centre field) and a calcified Michaelis–Gutmann body in the upper field on the left. These bodies probably represent the end result of incomplete lysosomal digestion of engulfed *E. coli*.

Lower tract pathology

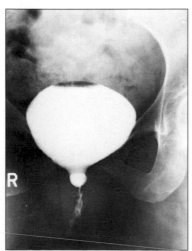

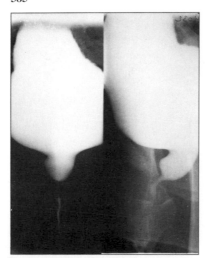

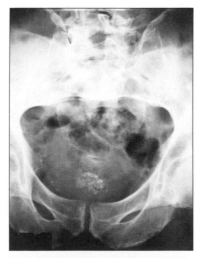

384, 385 Inflammatory disease of the female urethra may be associated with urethral stenosis, which is seen in this MCU.

386 Chronic prostatitis is usually abacterial, but chronic bacterial infection may occur in the presence of prostatic calculi. *Chlamydia* must be excluded.

Chyluria

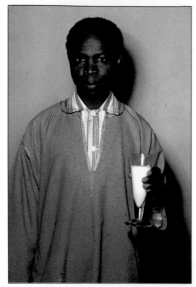

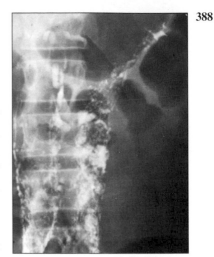

387 Chyluria. Milky urine as a result of the presence of chyle is rare except in patients from filarial-endemic areas. The parasite, *Wuchereria bancrofti,* invades the lymphatics and causes an inflammatory reaction, which results in obstruction. The parasite is a nematode. Mature helminths live in connective tissue and lymphatics. The microfilariae are released into the blood, usually at night. A wide variety of symptoms result but those seen in urology usually result from lymphatic obstruction. Megalymphatics that develop as a result may fistulate to the urinary tract and thus produce chyluria. Here a patient shows a specimen of milky urine.

388 Chyluria. Lymphangiogram studies show dye tracking towards the region of the left kidney.

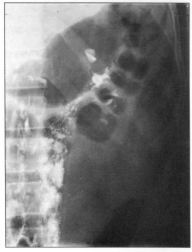

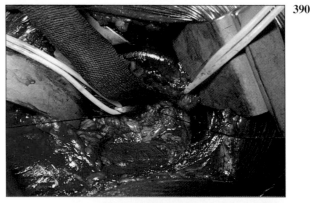

389 Chyluria. Later studies show well-outlined calyces, confirming a fistula.

390 Chyluria. Where these fistulae occur in the kidney megalymphatics may be found in the renal pedicle at exploration.

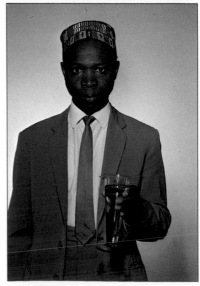

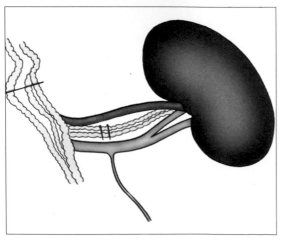

391 Parasitic chyluria. Diagram of megalymphatics. Points of ligations are shown.

392 Chyluria. Patient with a specimen of clear urine after lymphatic ligation. Rarely, the syndrome of chylous reflux in primary lymphoedema may produce chyluria as a result of obstruction in both megalymphatic syndrome and in lymphatic deficiency.

393

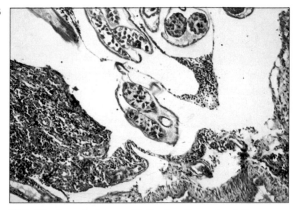

393 *Wuchereria bancrofti*. Section through adult worms (centre and upper field) with surrounding inflammatory reaction. *(H&E × 64)*

394

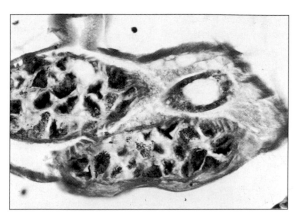

394 *Wuchereria bancrofti*. Higher magnification of section through an adult worm. *(H&E × 256)*

HIV and urology

Acquired immune-deficiency syndrome (AIDS), the terminal manifestation of human immunodeficiency virus (HIV) infection, was first recognised in 1981 and the causative virus was isolated two years later. The main mode of transmission is sexual, with anal intercourse being more efficient than vaginal. Spread also occurs through blood, blood products, and needle stick injury (although the risk of needle stick injury causing infection is less than 0.5%, HIV being approximately 100-fold less infectious than hepatitis B). In developing countries especially eastern Africa, high proportions of the hetero-sexually active population may be infected. In developed countries the infection is mainly among homosexual men, intravenous drug abusers, and their immediate sexual contacts. Heterosexual transmission does occur, but HIV is rarely found in individuals who are genuinely unaware of any risk.

The main effect of HIV is to deplete the immune system of T-helper lymphocytes. The process usually takes several years during which an individual remains asymptomatic. A test for HIV antibodies will however have become positive within three months of exposure in the majority of cases, and indicates persisting infection.

The immunosuppression is eventually manifest by opportunistic infections or tumours, such as *Pneumocystis carinii* pneumonia and Kaposi's sarcoma (KS). A small number of common infections are more severe in the presence of HIV, for example:

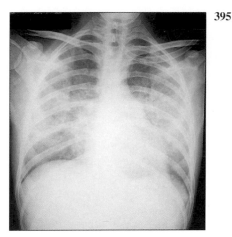

395 Typical *Pneumocystis carinii* pneumonia presenting with the radiographic features of an atypical pneumonia radiating from the hila.

- Severe chronic herpetic genital ulcers, which may be the presenting features of AIDS.
- Genital warts, which in the presence of HIV are strongly linked to intraepithelial neoplasia.
- Candidiasis.

These sexually transmitted diseases are also important

because their presence increases the likelihood of sexual transmission of HIV.

Generally HIV infection has few urological features, but in late disease when neuropathy is common, nocturia, with or without bacteriuria may be a problem. Other common conditions in AIDS such as KS, B-cell lymphoma, and *Mycobacterium tuberculosis* infection can occur at any site and occasionally affect the urogenital tract. KS is seen in about 20% of homosexuals with AIDS, but rarely in other groups, and is often found on the penis though

seldom as an isolated lesion. In terminal disease atypical mycobacteria are often disseminated and can be found in the urine, but this does not usually imply a local infection.

When contemplating an operative procedure it is important to be aware that thrombocytopenia can be associated with asymptomatic HIV infection. Most individuals with HIV are young and relatively resilient but appearances commonly deceive and as with other patients healing in terminal disease is often poor.

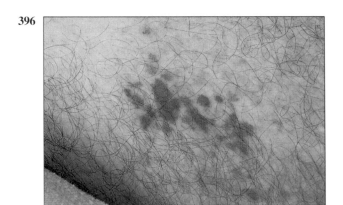

396 Typical purple skin eruption of Kaposi's sarcoma.

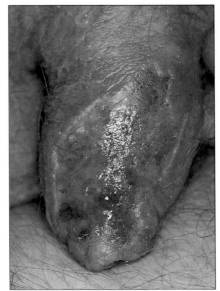

397 Erosive penile lesion of herpes in a patient with HIV infection.

4 Tuberculosis

Genitourinary tuberculosis is one manifestation of a systemic disease caused by the vascular metastatic spread of *Mycobacterium tuberculosis* from a primary focus, which is usually in the lung. It is a disease seen less and less in developed countries because of modern chemotherapy and better patient compliance, but still poses many problems in developing countries.

Presentation

The most common presentation of genitourinary tuberculosis is a young male with painless nocturia and increasing lack of energy, which may or may not be accompanied by diurnal frequency. Dysuria is uncommon, unless there is superimposed secondary infection. Haematuria is present in only approximately 8–10% of cases, and renal pain in 15–20%.

There are three important initial investigations:
● Radiology, not only of the renal tract but also of the chest, which might show scarring indicative of an original primary focus.

● Urine analysis, looking especially for sterile pyuria (i.e. 20 cells per 1/16th high power field), which is present in more than 70% of cases.
● Examination of three or more consecutive early morning specimens of urine to isolate *M. tuberculosis* and *M. bovis*. There are the organisms that cause tuberculosis, and both are acid- and alcohol-fast and nonmotile. However, they show differences in morphology. The human strain is slender, and slightly curved, and the bovine strain is straight and stubby, and occurs singly or in pairs.

Investigations

Intravenous urography

The intravenous urogram (IVU) is still the first and most important interpretation in this condition because the calcyceal changes can be very small. Ultrasound may have a role in assessing the progress of more advanced lesions.

The initial lesion occurs in the parenchyma of the kidney close to a glomerulus and spreads immediately to involve the collecting system, producing tubercle bacilli in the urine. These lesions expand and produce the many different changes seen on the IVU.

Any tuberculous infection is of two types:
● A fulminating acute process, with poor host resistance, which causes the ulcerocavernous lesion and destruction of renal tissue.
● A more benign lesion caused by a less virulent organism which, together with more effective host resistance, results in a slowly growing fibrotic type of disease.

398

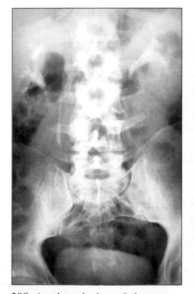

398 A minor lesion of the upper pole of the right kidney. Note the disorganisation of the upper calyx.

399

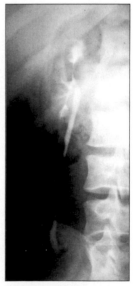

399 Same lesion, oblique view. The extent of the lesion is more easily seen.

400

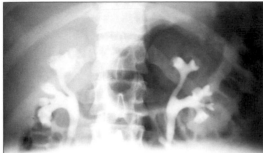

400 A minor lesion of the upper pole of the right kidney, becoming more invasive. In this patient the disease had spread to affect more than one calyx, which had become irregular and deformed with papillary cavitation.

401

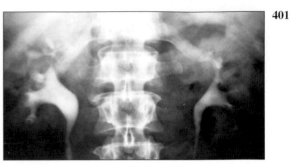

401 Typical trifoliate lesion of the upper pole of the right kidney. This is a more advanced lesion, in which the disease has involved the neck of the calyx, which then becomes constricted, resulting in the classical cicatrical appearance.

402

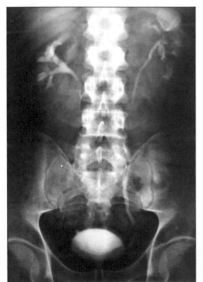

402 Ulcerocavernous disease. The disease has progressed and renal substance has been destroyed. Note that the damage is closely related to a calyx, and that the cortical thickness remains unchanged, but the cavity involves both renal tissue and the calyceal system.

403

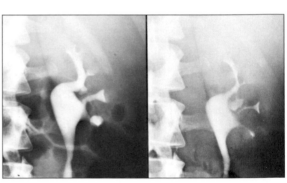

403 Solitary ulcerocavernous lesion in the middle calyx; this is a rare manifestation.

404

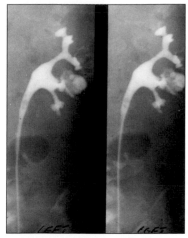

404 A more advanced middle caly-ceal lesion, which is only shown on retrograde pyelogram. This is an investigation which is now rarely required because an IVU nearly always supplies all the vital information. Nevertheless it cannot be abandoned completely.

405

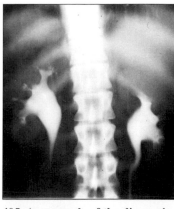

405 An example of the disease in-volving multiple calyces, but show-ing minimal parenchymal damage, again emphasising that cortical invol-vement is a very late phenomenon.

406

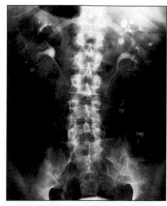

406 Another example of a more advanced disease involving multiple calyces. This shows more parenchymal damage, but the renal function is good. This type of lesion is usually of many years' duration and is caused by organ-isms of low virulence.

407

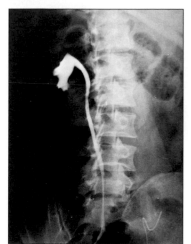

407 Extensive low grade disease, causing fibrosis of the calyceal stem, so that the area of the kidney that drains into the diseased calyceal system ceases to function and on urography gives the typical cut-off appearance.

408

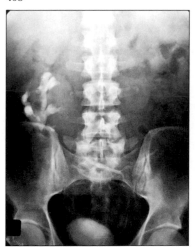

408 A moderate lesion affecting one half of a horseshoe kidney. Congen-itally abnormal kidneys are rarely affected by the mycobacterium.

409

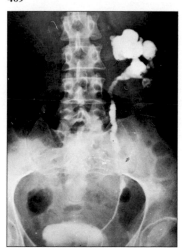

409 An example of unilateral ex-tensive disease.

410

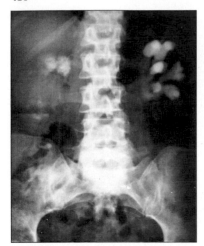

411

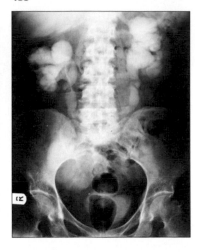

410, 411 Bilateral extensive disease. In the type of lesion shown the disease has progressed to destroy a large part of functioning renal tissue, resulting in a disorganised pelviureteric system, with cavities in the renal parenchyma.

412

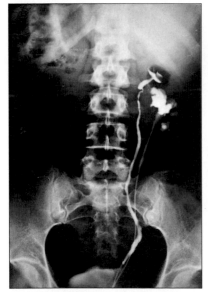

413

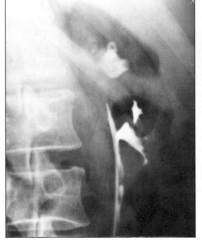

414

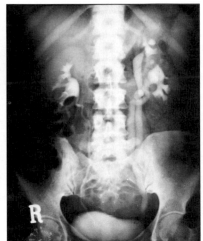

412 Occasionally, renal tuberculosis affects one moiety of a duplex system, as in this example.

413 A lateral view of renal tuberculosis affecting one moiety of a duplex system. This outlines the lesion in greater detail.

414 Example of renal tuberculosis involving both moieties of a duplex kidney, which is a very rare manifestation.

Macroscopic appearance

415 Gross renal tuberculosis, showing almost complete destruction of renal tissue. The cortex is thinned and there are numerous cavities. This is the end result of long-standing disease.

416 Complete destruction of the kidney by tuberculosis.

417 Radiograph showing calcification in this caseous pyonephrosis.

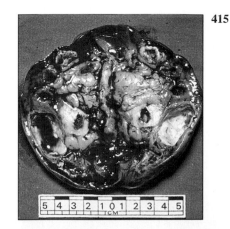
415

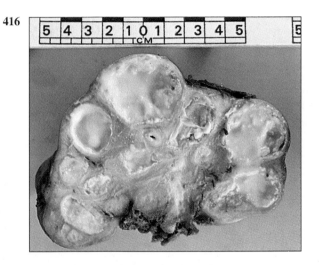
416

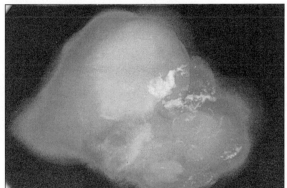
417

Histology

418 Renal tuberculosis. In the bottom right corner of the picture is a glomerulus. In the centre and upper left hand side of the picture is a giant cell granuloma. This is composed of a central zone of histiocytic cells derived from monocytes in the blood, some of which have become epithelioid in appearance (i.e. their plentiful cytoplasm has become eosinophilic and they resemble squamous cells). Other have fused to form a multinuclear giant cell, which has its nuclei arranged around the periphery of the cell (i.e. it is a Langhan's type giant cell). Around the periphery of the granuloma there are lymphocytes and plasma cells. This granuloma is in the cortex of the kidney. It has not yet undergone the central necrosis, which is seen as caseation in older granulomas. *(H&E × 160)*

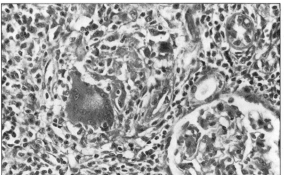
418

419

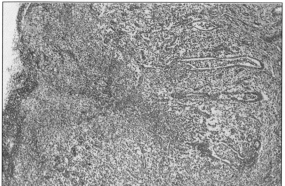

420

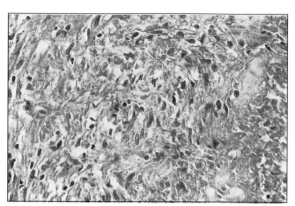

419 Renal tuberculosis. In the medulla there is widespread infiltration with chronic inflammatory cells, and the tubules are being destroyed. There is necrosis and the papilla is undergoing necrosis. There is a ragged edge on the left hand side of the picture. (H&E x 160)

420 Renal tuberculosis. A long-standing lesion. Some necrosis is evident at the right hand side. In most of the field there is plentiful eosinophilic collagen, being laid down by fibroblasts replacing the inflammatory cells. This fibrosis is common around old tuberculous lesions, and often calcifies.

Calcification

Calcification is important because 50–60% of patients have a calcified lesion somewhere in the renal tract when first seen. If present, investigations are the same as for patients with a renal tract calculus. The calcified lesion varies from a small discrete area in the kidney to involving all parts of the urinary system and appears to be of two types: progressive and static. It is impossible to tell whether it will progress and damage the kidney or remain unchanged for years; hence the danger and importance of following up such patients indefinitely.

The importance of tuberculous renal calcification has been highlighted because of the increasing use of the litho-triptor for treating renal calculi. Recently two cases of miliary tuberculosis have been recorded following the treatment of renal calculi by the lithotriptor. It is therefore important to exclude a history of renal tuberculosis before using this method of treatment for calculi. These cases of miliary tuberculosis are not surprising because 30% of tuberculosis calcification harbours viable *M. tuberculosis* in the calcified matrix.

421

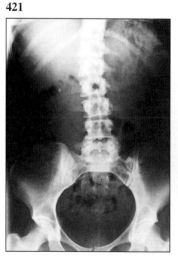

422

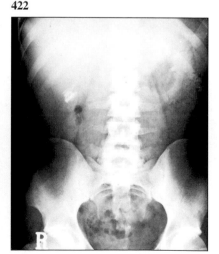

423

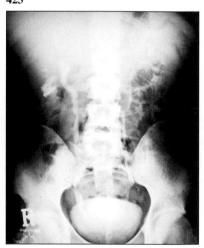

421 Small, discrete renal calculus, plain urogram. It is impossible to distinguish this from a solitary renal calculus, until *M. tuberculosis* is isolated from the urine.

422, 423 Larger area plain urogram and IVU. A progressive type, which usually involves either the upper or lower pole.

424   425

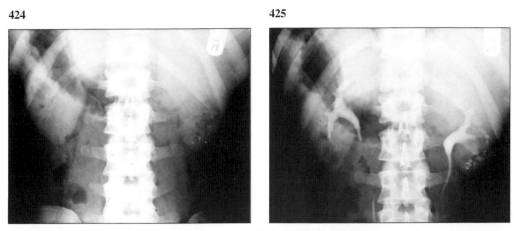

424, 425 Another larger area, plain film and IVU. This is an unusual presentation because it simulates nephrocalcinosis with minimal parenchymal damage. The lesion can not be confirmed until mycobacterium are isolated from the urine.

426   427   428

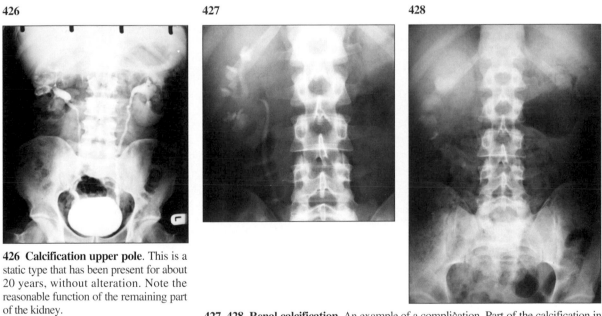

426 Calcification upper pole. This is a static type that has been present for about 20 years, without alteration. Note the reasonable function of the remaining part of the kidney.

427, 428 Renal calcification. An example of a complication. Part of the calcification in the lower pole of a solitary kidney has become detached, causing an almost total ureteric obstruction. IVU appearance before and after ureteric obstruction.

Progressive calcification

Progressive calcification can spread slowly and insidiously, and may take many years to destroy the kidney.

429   **430**   **431**

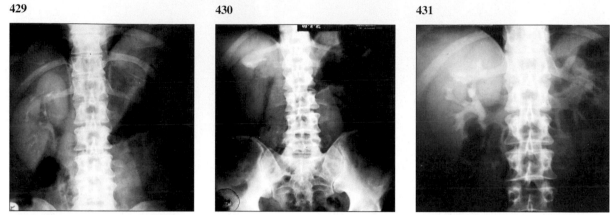

429, 430, 431 Progressive calcification affecting the upper pole of a solitary kidney. 429 shows minimal calcification with scarring. **430** and **431** show the plain film and IVU appearances 1 year later.

432

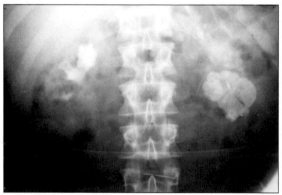

433

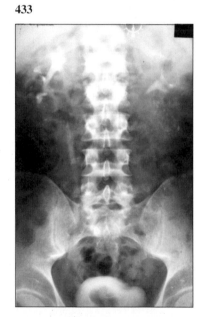

432, 433, 434, 435, 436 Another example of what can happen if patients with calcification are not adequately supervised. This patient had a cavernotomy for a calcified lesion in the lower pole of the left kidney. The pathology in the right kidney was not considered severe enough to warrant careful supervision. **432** shows the condition before left cavernotomy. **433** shows the condition one year later; there is diffuse calcification in the lower pole of the right kidney. **434** one year later shows that the calcification is denser, and in **435** a further year later the spread and density of the calcification has increased. In **436,** 1 year later, two-thirds of the kidney have been destroyed by slowly progressive calcification. *M. tuberculosi*s was never isolated from this patient, and on histological examination the section shows chronic pyelonephritis with diffuse parenchymal calcification.

434

435

436

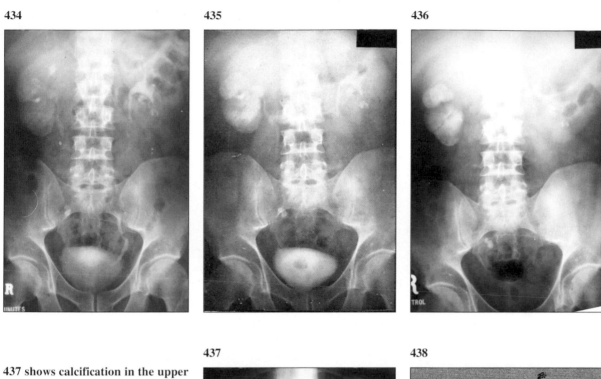

437

438

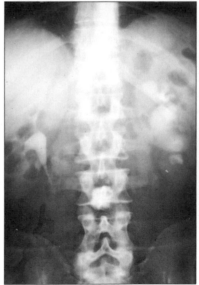

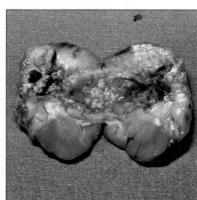

437 shows calcification in the upper pole with active disease and hydro-nephrosis. 438 shows calcification with active caseating disease. In this resected upper pole specimen, the calcification is shown in the middle of an area in which the renal parenchyma has been destroyed. This is a progressive type of disease and it is in this type of lesion that a selective renal arteriogram may help to decide the amount of tissue to be excised because invariably there is more renal damage than is shown on an IVU.

439

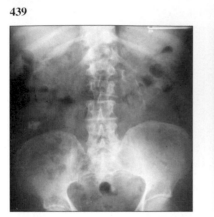

440

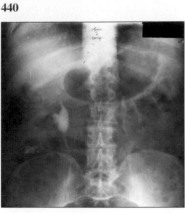

441

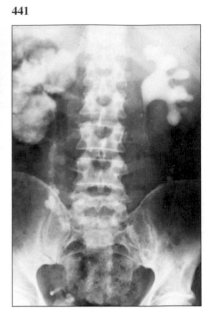

439, 440, 441 The calcified kidney may be contracted and situated over the psoas muscle, and may be difficult to differentiate from a calcified psoas abscess without an IVU. However, if the latter is the cause of the calcification, destructive changes in the vertebra should be excluded. It is essential to X-ray the thoracic as well as the dorsal spine because the abscess may track down from the thoracic region before entering the region of the psoas muscle. **439** Plain film with calcified shadow over the psoas muscle. **440** An IVU reveals a nonfunctioning left kidney. **441** Plain urogram with calcification involving one kidney, the ureter, seminal vesicles, and the prostate.

Tuberculosis of the ureter

Tuberculosis of the ureter can cause strictures in the pelviureteric junction, in the middle third of the ureter, and at the ureterovesical junction. The commonest site is the ureterovesical junction, where it occurs in about 9% of cases.

442

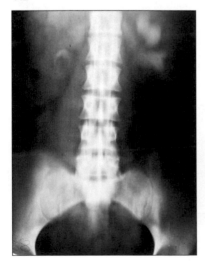

443

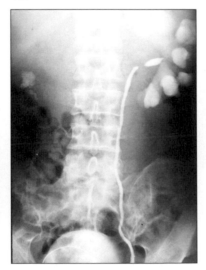

442 Stricture at the pelviureteric junction. This is a rare manifestation, because the combination of acute virulent infection with obstruction of the pelviureteric junction destroys the kidney before treatment can be started. Nevertheless, when diagnosed, the treatment must be immediate and aggressive to relieve the obstruction. It should always be carried out under antituberculous chemotherapy cover.

443 Two strictures. Another rare manifestation, involving the pelvis, causing obstruction at the pelvicalyceal junction of all the calyceal systems. This condition poses great problems in treatment, especially if the kidney is solitary.

Strictures of the middle third of
the ureter are very rare, but if seen
early enough, can be effectively
treated.

**444 Stricture of the middle third of
the ureter** treated by prolonged
ureteric catheterisation with a silastic
tube.

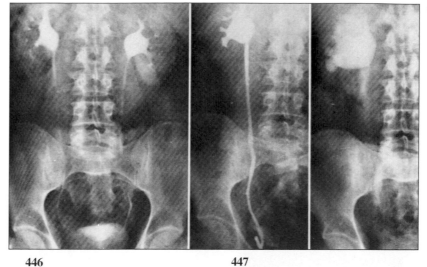

444

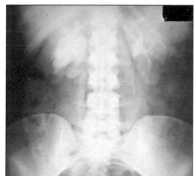

445

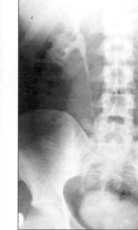

446

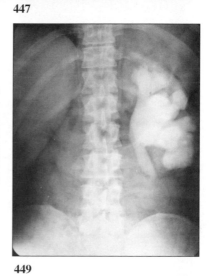

447

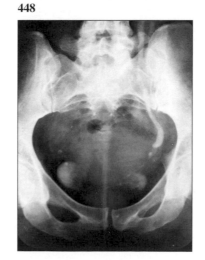

448

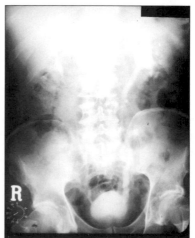

449

**445 Stricture of the upper third of the
ureter** with hydronephrosis, a very rare
manifestation.

**446 Stricture at the lower end of the
ureter,** with dilatation of the whole of the
upper urinary tract. Strictures at the lower
end of the ureter are caused by fibrosis.

**447 A more advanced stricture of the
lower end of the ureter**, in which the
hydronephrosis is more pronounced.

**448 Stricture of the lower end of a
bifid system**.

**449 Stricture of the pelviureteric
junction and at the ureterovesical
junction**. Strictures may be multiple, but
this is a very rare manifestation. It is
more usual to find the whole of the ureter
replaced by fibrous tissue.

450

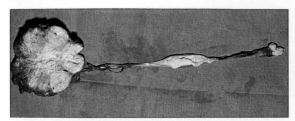

450 A kidney completely destroyed by a combination of strictures at the pelviureteric junction, the middle third of the ureter, and at the ureterovesical junction.

451

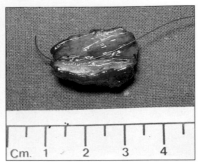

451 Specimen of excised ureterovesical stricture, showing fibrosis, oedema and a narrow lumen. The disease in this patient had advanced beyond the reach of conservative treatment, and early surgery was mandatory.

452

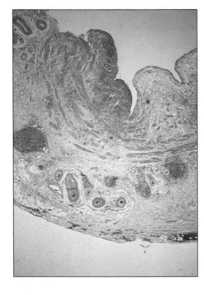

453

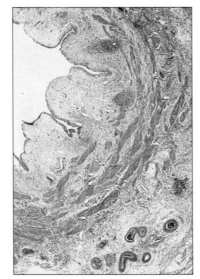

452 Microscopic appearance of 451. Ureter showing chronic inflammatory cells extending right through the wall and fibrosis occurring in all coats. The mucosa is oedematous, and underlying bands of muscle are separated. Inflammatory cells are scattered through the wall and aggregated into groups.

453 Histological appearance of the same ureter as shown in 451 and 452, stained with trichrome and showing extensive fibrous infiltration.

454

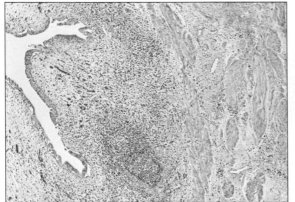

454 Fibrous tissue separating the muscle bands and involving the mucosa. Lymphoid aggregates are seen, but there are no granulomas.

455

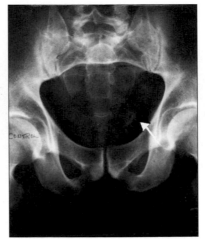

A calcified stricture at the lower end of the ureter causing almost complete obstruction is a very rare finding.

455 A plain film of such a ureter.

456 IVU showing hydronephrosis and poor renal function.

457 Specimen showing calcification and a thickened fibrous ureter.

458 Histological appearance of calcification after total decalcification, showing caseous material in the upper left hand side of the field.

459 Ziehl-Nielsen stain of amorphous tissue after treatment, showing clumps of degenerate bacilli.

456

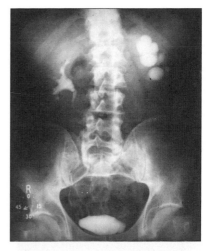

457

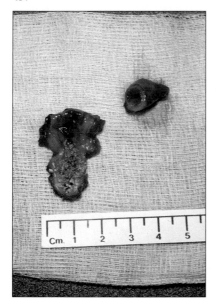

458

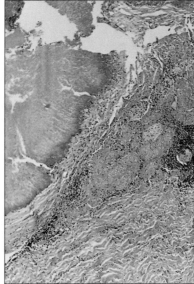

459

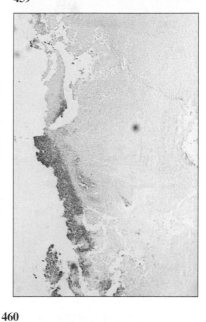

460

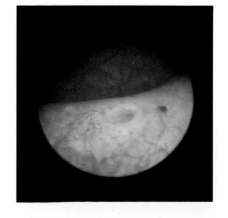

Endoscopy

Tuberculous cystitis presents in many ways, but always starts with a mild inflammation around a tuberculous ureteric orifice. It can spread and involve the whole bladder, producing an intense, diffuse cystitis.

460 Tuberculous cystitis: a mild infection. The orifice is oedematous and beginning to gape. Every case of tuberculous cystitis starts at the ureteric orifice.

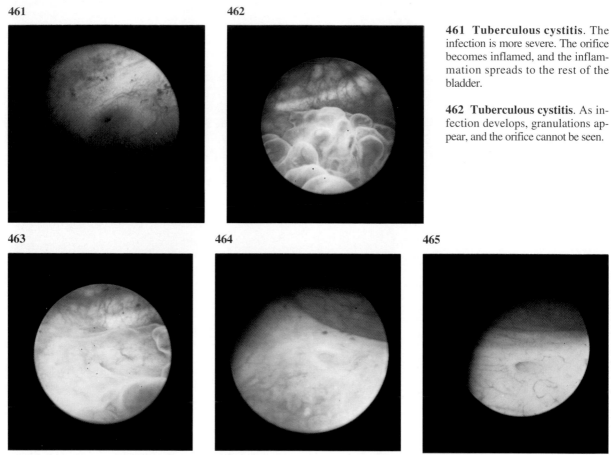

461 Tuberculous cystitis. The infection is more severe. The orifice becomes inflamed, and the inflammation spreads to the rest of the bladder.

462 Tuberculous cystitis. As infection develops, granulations appear, and the orifice cannot be seen.

463, 464, 465 Tuberculous cystitis. As healing progresses, the granulations disappear and the orifice can then be seen. Ultimately the orifice can return almost to normal, but appears pale (**464**), and indrawn (**465**).

Golf-hole ureter

In a severe infection, granulations completely cover the ureteric orifice, and it cannot be seen. The granulations may slowly disappear, leaving an inflamed oedematous orifice. In cases that respond rapidly to modern chemo- therapy, the orifice ultimately looks scarred. In more long-standing cases the ureter becomes indrawn, producing the classic golf-hole appearance. This can be clear-cut or surrounded by fibrous tissue.

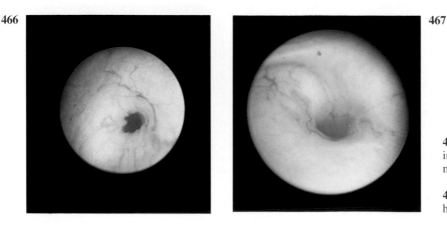

466 Small golf-hole ureter. It is irregular, and the surrounding mucous membrane is pale and atrophic.

467 Golf-hole ureter, which is a rigid, healed orifice.

110

468

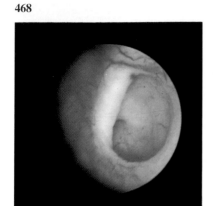

468 Golf-hole ureter on the floor of a false diverticulum.

469

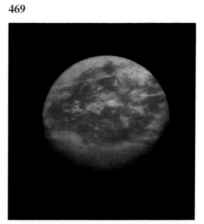

469 Tuberculous ulcer showing central slough.

470

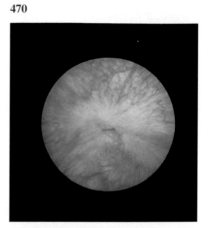

470 Healed cystitis scar. As the cystitis heals it produces a scar, often of stellate form, very similar to that of a Hunner's ulcer.

471

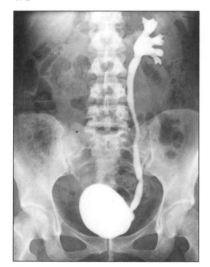

471 Tuberculous cystitis with strictures at the lower end of the ureter, showing a contracted bladder.

472

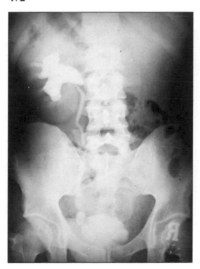

472 IVU of advanced tuberculous cystitis, with stricture of the lower end of the ureter, showing a contracted bladder.

473

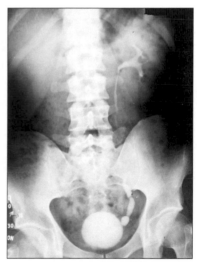

473 Early tuberculous cystitis and an early ureteric stricture. The urographic appearances of the kidney are normal.

Tuberculosis of the seminal vesicles

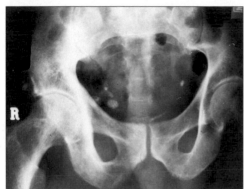

474

Tuberculosis of the seminal vesicles is rare and is nearly always associated with tuberculous prostatitis and epididymitis. When the acute phase heals, calcification is common.

474 Plain film showing calcification of the seminal vesicles.

Tuberculous prostatitis

Tuberculous prostatitis is particularly common in association with tuberculosis of the epididymis, which often contains calculi.

475

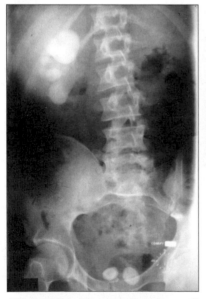

476

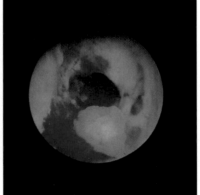

476 Endoscopic view of tuberculous prostatitis showing the cavity from which the calculus has been extruded.

477

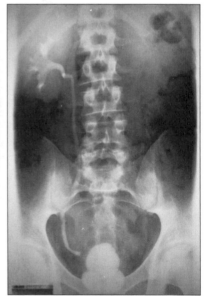

475 Calculi in the prostate with a small contracted bladder and hydronephrosis of a solitary kidney.

477 Large prostatic cavities caused by destruction of the prostate.

Generalised tuberculosis of the urinary tract

On rare occasions, infection may involve all parts of the urinary tract and pose severe problems in management.

478 **Tuberculous cystitis** combined with a stricture of the lower end of the ureter and tuberculous prostatic cavitation.

478

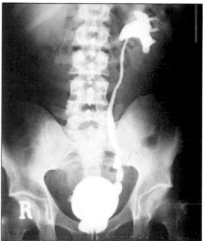

479

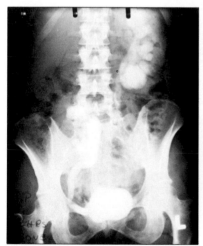

480

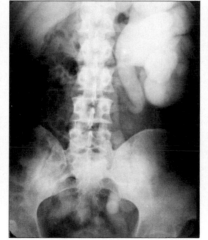

481

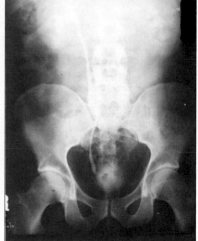

479 Tuberculous left kidney, bladder, and right ectopic kidney.

480 Severe renal tuberculosis of a solitary kidney with ureteric reflux and a small contracted bladder.

481 Severe left renal tuberculosis with a small contracted bladder and an early stricture of the right ureter.

Urethral strictures

Tuberculous urethral stricture is rare, and once the acute infection is under control it should be managed in the same way as any other inflammatory stricture. On urography it is indistinguishable from other urethral strictures.

482

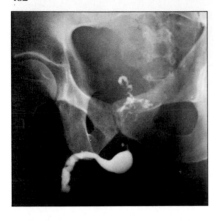

483

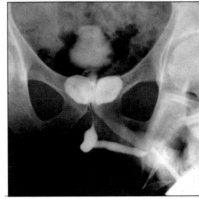

482 Ascending urethrogram of a tuberculous urethral stricture.

483 Ascending urethrogram of a tuberculous urethral stricture with a small contracted bladder, prostatic cavitation and perineal fistula.

Tuberculous epididymitis

Tuberculous epididymitis is a common presenting sign. The patient first complains of a painful scrotal swelling, which may or may not be accompanied by a disturbance of micturition. Tuberculosis of the testis is always secondary to tuberculosis of the epididymis.

484

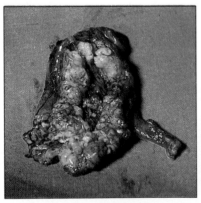

484 Tuberculous epididymitis.

485

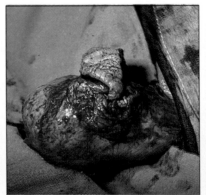

485 Tuberculous epididymitis with a skin lesion.

486

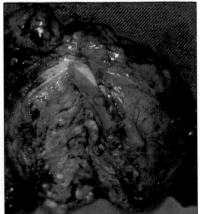

486 Tuberculous epididymitis involving the testis, which occurs in 5% of cases of tuberculous epididymitis.

5 Schistosomiasis (bilharziasis) of the genitourinary system

Bilharziasis is a disease found in many parts of the world, but is mainly endemic in the greater part of Africa. The main species causing disease in man are *Schistosoma haematobium*, which predominantly affects the urinary tract, and *S. mansoni* and *S. japonicum*, which cause intestinal disease. *S. haematobium* is a trematode. The adult male is 10–15 mm long and 2 mm broad and has two suckers anteriorly. Its body is irregularly covered with round projections and together with the suckers these help to anchor the worm to the venous wall of the host. The female is 8–17 mm long and 1 mm wide and lies enclosed in the gynaecophoric canal of the male.

487

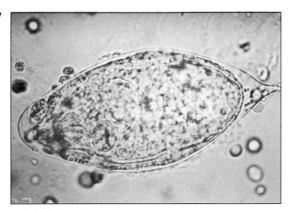

487 Egg in the urine. The eggs are oval and about 120 mm in length. The shell has a distinct terminal spine. *S. mansoni* has a subterminal spine, and the embryo is visible within. When the infected urine becomes diluted on being mixed with water the shell swells and bursts and a ciliated embryo or miracidium escapes.

488

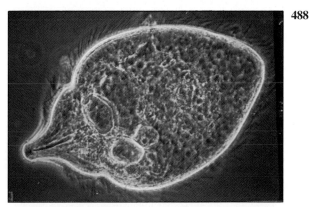

488 Ciliated miracidium. The miracidium swims actively, searching for the intermediate hosts, the *Bulinus contortus*, a freshwater snail. When encountered it is penetrated by the miracidia, which eventually reach the liver where they develop into cercariae, forming multiple hepatic sporocysts.

489

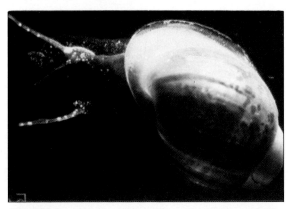

489 *Bulinus contortus*. After about a month the snail dies and the ovocysts rupture and discharge thousands of cercariae into the water.

490

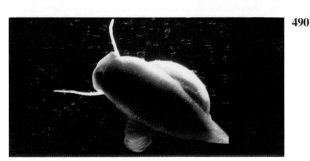

490 *Bulinus contortus* discharging cercariae.

491

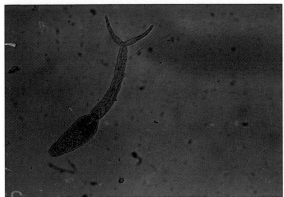

491 Cerceriae are 2 mm long with a pear-shaped head and a bifid tail. They infect their definitive host, usually man, chiefly through the skin but also through the mucous membrane of the mouth and pharynx. The cerceria leaves its tail during penetration of the skin.

492

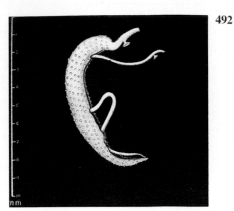

492 Male worm with a female in the gynaecophoric canal.

493

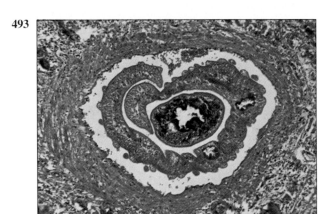

493 Adult schistosomes. The female lies enfolded in the gynaecophoric grooves of the male. They are both inside a small vein in the bladder wall. Some eggs and inflammation are seen in the surrounding tissues. *(H&E × 80)*

494

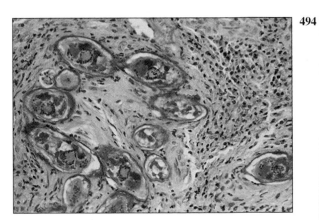

494 Eggs in perivenous tissue. These elicit an inflammatory reaction, which may be very variable in its pattern. *(Periodic acid Schiff × 256)*

495

496

497

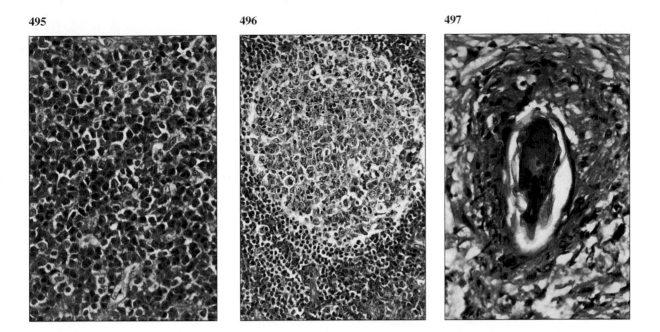

495 Schistosomiasis. Inflammation in the bladder wall. Here there is a very heavy infiltrate of eosinophils, with other inflammatory cells. *(H&E × 256)*

496 Schistosomiasis. Inflammation in the bladder wall. Occasionally lymphoid follicles with reactive centres form. *(H&E × 160)*

497 Schistosomiasis. Inflammation in the bladder wall showing some histiocytes surrounding an ovum. There is fibrosis around the histiocytes. *(H&E × 256)*

498 Detailed schematic drawing of the life cycle of *S. haematobium* as it affects man. In the bladder the area that appears to be the portal of entry of bilharzia is known as the 'Magarr', which is the Arabic word for the 'Milky Way'. This Magarr area extends from the right side of the bladder below the air bubble to cross the midline to the left side of the bladder. Here it assumes a more or less vertical direction, which it maintains to about 3.5 cm above and to the left of the left ureteric orifice. Then it crosses the midline again to end about 2.5 cm above and to the right of the right ureteric orifice. The Magarr area is at the junction of the fixed and mobile parts of the bladder, where it is richly supplied with blood. This area of the posterior and superior walls is supplied by one vessel, the superior vesical artery. In the bladder during the early stages of bilharzial infestation, there is patchy congestion due to acute mucosal hyperaemia.

498

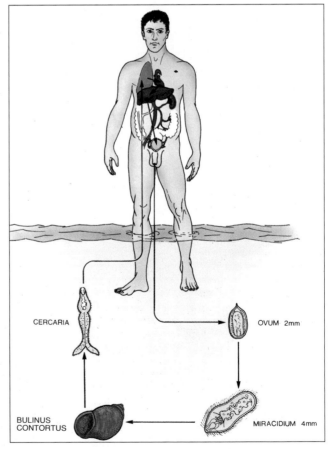

CERCARIA

OVUM 2mm

BULINUS CONTORTUS

MIRACIDIUM 4mm

499

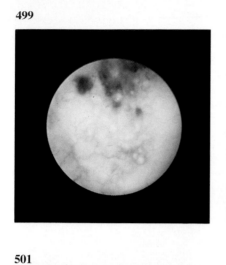

500

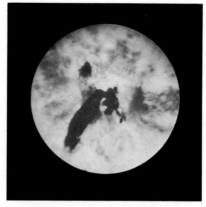

499, 500 Cystoscopic appearance of the earliest acute bilharzial lesions in the bladder.

501

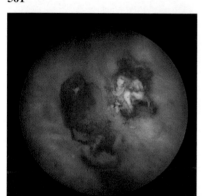

502

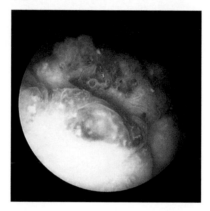

501 Active bilharzial cystitis with flat granuloma and stelate ulcer.

502 Active bilharzial cystitis. The mucosa is thrown into polypoid folds with oedema and granulation.

503

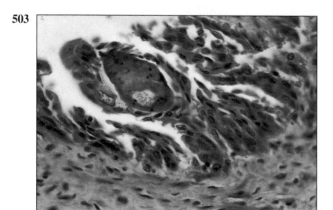

504

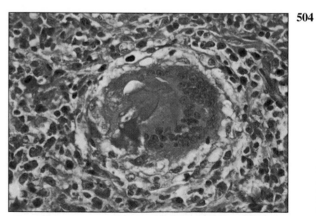

503 Bladder mucosa showing a schistosoma egg passing through epithelium into the bladder lumen. *(H&E × 256)*

504 Bladder wall showing granuloma formation in response to the presence of eggs. Some of the histiocytes have fused to form a multinucleate giant cell. *(H&E × 256)*

505 Bladder wall showing dead ova with very little inflammatory reaction. The pink staining material is fibrous tissue. This would appear as a sandy patch on endoscopy. *(H&E × 160)*

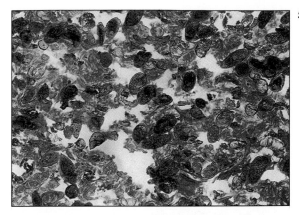

505

506

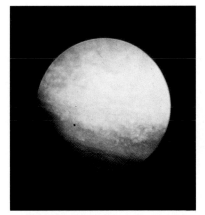

507

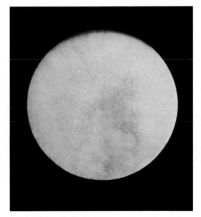

508

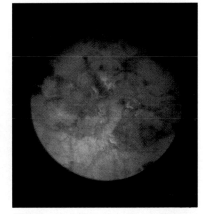

506 A sandy patch. This is caused by a mucosal reaction to submucosal ova deposition, in which whole layers of epithelium except basement membrane are shed. The ova appear as packed sand under water and the areas are pale brown. Dead and calcified ova are deposited under wider areas of the mucosa and look as white as sheets.

507 Ground-glass mucosa. On other occasions the bladder mucosa can ulcerate and become infected.

508 Septic bilharzial ulcers. The rest of the vesical mucosa shows signs of inflammation.

509

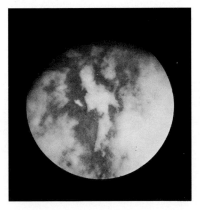

510

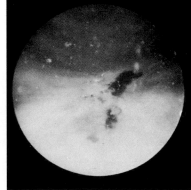

509 Chronic superficial ulcer. This is larger than an acute ulcer. It has irregular edges and a pale anaemic floor surrounded by congested hyperaemic mucous membrane.

510 Chronic deep ulcer. Bilharzial tubercles on top, and ground-glass mucosa below.

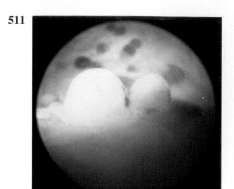

511 **Bilharzial cystitis cystica**.

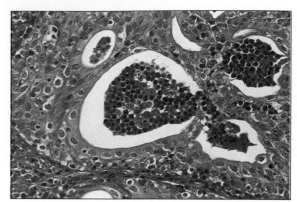

512 **Cystitis cystica** showing cystic spaces lined with transitional epithelium and inflammation. Occasionally the epithelium shows a glandular metaplasia and the condition is then called cystitis glandularis. *(H&E × 160)*

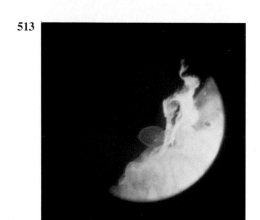

513 **Chronic deep ulcer**. Bilharzial tubercles above, ground-glass mucosa below. Ulcers show complete denudation of the mucosa including the basement membrane. The base of this lesion comprises granulation or fibrous tissue according to the stage of the ulcer, which may be acute or chronic. Chronic ulcers may be superficial, deep, or stellate. Bilharzial ulcers never turn malignant.

The bladder mucosa may react more actively, producing hyperplastic lesions such as cystitis cystica, cystitis glanularis, bilharzial polypi, or malignant neoplasms.

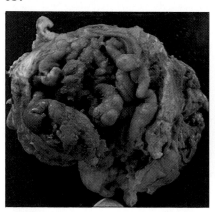

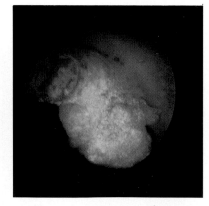

514 **Bladder schistosomiasis**. This bladder shows marked thickening, with the mucosa thrown up into polypoid folds.

515 **Giant bilharzial granuloma**. The condition goes on to form giant bilharzial granuloma.

516

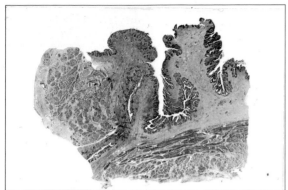

517

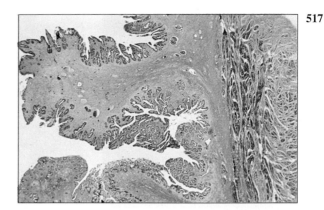

518

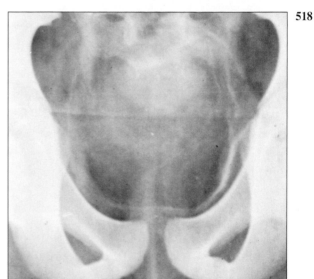

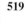

519

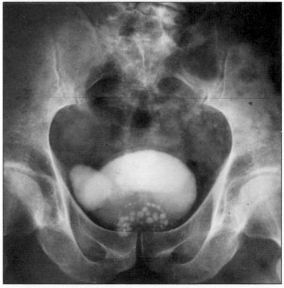

516 Bladder schistosomiasis. Section through the wall of **514** showing the mucosa with polyp formation. The epithelium is hyperplastic and covers cores of connective tissue. No neoplasm was present despite its florid appearances. *(H&E original section, life size)*

517 Bladder schistosomiasis. Similar section to **516** but stained with a trichrome to show the fibrous tissue (green). *(Trichrome × 31)*

Radiologically these two conditions show as filling defects on urograms. When urinary crystalloids are deposited on the ruptured cysts, they appear as calcified shadows on plain radiography.

Bilharzial infection of bladder muscle has three stages: irritable bladder; weak bladder; contracted bladder.

518 IVU of bilharzial calcification of the bladder wall. The bladder is distended and its upper border has reached the sacroiliac joint. This is the stage of bladder irritability before that of acute fibrosis. The muscle wall may be hypertrophied or at least spastic in the irritative phase of acute infiltration. The bladder wall is then thicker and may produce temporary pressure on the intravesical ureter, while the ureter itself, continuing to contract, may cause noncalcular renal colic or temporary back pressure on the upper parts of the ureter or even the kidney.

In the weak stage, mild muscle fibrosis interferes with the power of bladder contractility. Further fibrosis causes dilatation and thinning of the wall and formation of a retrotrigonal pouch.

519 Bladder neck obstruction with a diverticulum in the right lateral wall and mutiple calculi in the retrotrigonal pouch. This either alone or with an associated bladder neck fibrosis resembles an elevated bladder neck. This may resolve with treatment or may proceed to a stage in which there is residual urine due to dynamic atony as well as stenosis of the bladder neck. Finally contraction of the fibrous tissue is common and may be localised in the bladder neck, giving the syndrome of bladder neck fibrosis.

520

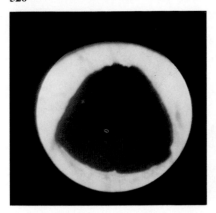

521

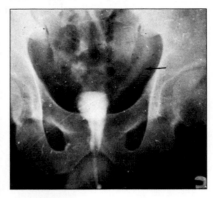

520 Endoscopic view of bladder neck fibrosis. The disease may affect the Magarr line and produce a bipartite bladder or it may affect the whole organ and produce a contracted bladder.

521 Cystogram showing a severely contracted bladder. The bladder may change from the normal to the hypertrophic thick-walled state, then dilate again to retrieve its normal size, proceeding further to the dilated atonic bladder, only to recontract again, leading to a useless scarred noncontractile contracted bladder.

Calcification is a classical finding in longstanding bilharzial disease of the urinary tract. Not only the bladder and bladder neck, but also the ureters, may be involved.

522

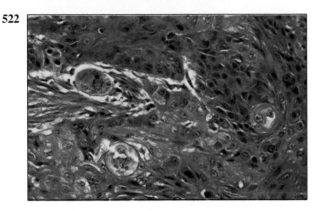

522 Carcinoma of the bladder occurs in association with schistomiasis. About 67% are squamous-type and may be related to squamous metaplasia occurring with the inflammation. About 25% are transitional-type, while the rest are adenocarcinomas. This section shows a squamous carcinoma with some associated eggs. *(H&E × 160)*

Radiological appearance of bilharzial bladder

523

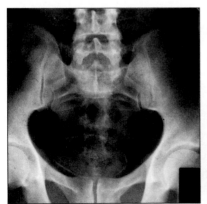

523 Plain radiograph of bilharzial calcified contracted bladder.

524

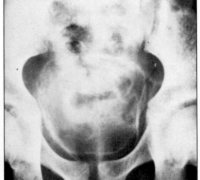

524 Plain radiograph of laminated calcification of bilharzial bladder, which also shows calcified dilated ureters with ureteritis calcinosa (calcified ureteritis cystica). An elevated and calcified base of bladder, typical of bilharzial bladder neck fibrosis, is also seen.

525

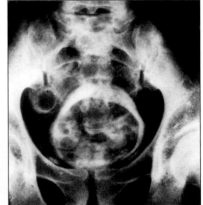

525 Plain radiograph of more advanced linear calcification of a dilated bladder with calcified base of bilharzial bladder neck fibrosis.

526

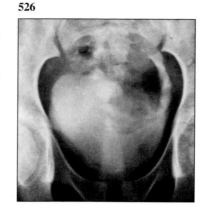

527

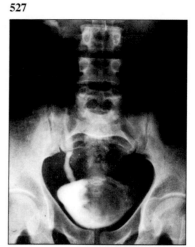

526 Plain radiograph showing disappearance of calcification on the left side of the bladder due to carcinoma of the bladder.

527 IVU showing the line of calcification on the left side, which is interrupted by the tumour tissue.

After cystoscopy, as an important means of studying the pathology of vesical bilharziasis, comes radiography. Plain radiography reveals hardly any bilharzial lesions before calcification. The appearance depends on the severity of calcification and density of fibrosis in the bladder wall. In mild cases linear shadows of calcification of the bladder wall are visible. In more advanced cases, there is laminated calcification of the bladder wall. In severe cases the vesical shadow forms a small circle or sphere, and the cavity of the bladder fills with irregular opacities.

Distortion and dissolution of calcification can occur in malignancy.

Bilharziasis of the ureter

In bilharziasis of the ureter the initial and subsequent pathology is the same as in the bladder. The commonest regions affected are the intramural part, which is usually involved secondary to bladder pathology, and then the juxtavesical part. Bilharzial changes in the ureter are almost always bilateral, but one ureter may be affected more than the other. The final result of the bilharzial infiltration of the ureter is dense fibrosis involving all or most of its layers; calcification is common.

528

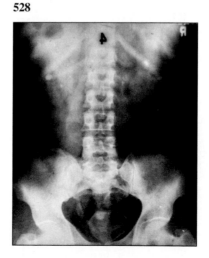

529

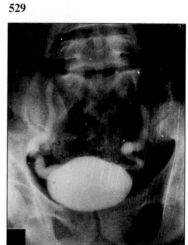

528 Plain radiograph showing a contracted and calcified bladder with a calcified right ureter and a stone in the right kidney. In mild fibrosis diminution of tone will cause the ureter to dilate in front of the pressure head of urine from the kidney, producing the typical spindle-shaped ureter of bilharziasis.

529 Early intramural bilharzial infection of the ureters leading to an intramural stricture and spindle-shaped dilatation of the ureter, especially of the left side.

123

530

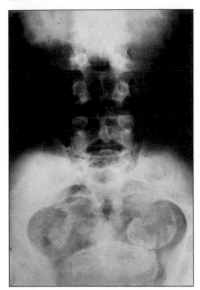

531

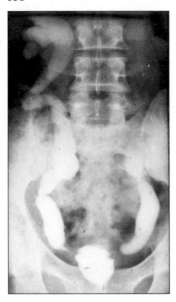

530 Plain radiograph of more advanced disease with calcification of the bladder and bilateral spindle-shaped dilated and calcified ureters. When fibrosis proceeds further it causes dilatation and tortuosity of the ureter, which assumes a small intestine-like appearance.

531 IVU showing a severely contracted and irregular bladder, severely constricted juxta-vesical parts of both ureters, and huge dilated elongated and tortuous intestine-like ureters with hydronephrosis. Contraction of the fibrous tissue also produces a stricture of the ureter at any level, usually in its lower third, but may be at the level of the third lumbar transverse process, with consequent proximal dilatation and tortuosity and with back pressure on the corresponding kidney.

Perivesical and periureteric fibrolipomatosis infiltration may press on the ureter from outside, adding to the ureteric obstruction and proximal dilatation.

Bilharzial ureteric reflux

532

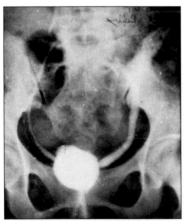

533

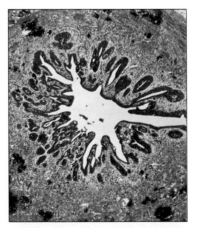

534

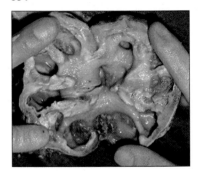

534 Infected hydronephrotic kidney with multiple big calculi in most of its pelvicalyceal system.

532 Ascending cystogram with grade II ureteric reflux. About 96% of cases of bilharzial ureteric reflux result from bladder neck fibrosis; infection is present in about 84%. Once reflux becomes established, progressive renal destruction usually follows, particularly in the presence of infection. Persistently severe bilateral reflux causes coarse scarring and back pressure atrophy of the kidney. Calcification is a secondary effect.

533 Ureter: schistosomiasis. A ureter with hyperplastic epithelium, thickened wall, and some calcified ova, which are almost black and seen at the top and bottom of the field. *(H&E × 26)*

535 Infected hydronephrotic kidney, ureteritis cystica and calcinosis. Note the unhealthy, thick, dilated ureter with ureteritis cystica.

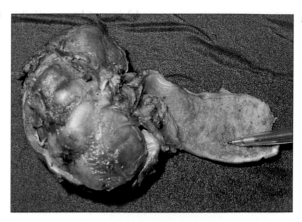

Bilharziasis of the urethra

Urethral bilharziasis is usually associated with vesical and urethral infection. The portal of entry of infection is through the deep dorsal vein of the penis from the pelvic pool of veins. The posterior urethral involvement is a part of bladder neck pathology giving congestion, hyperaemia, mild fibrosis and, rarely, ulcers.

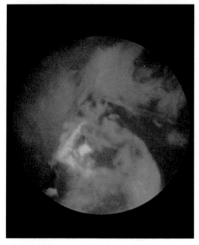

536 Urethroscopic view of bilharziasis of posterior urethra with ulcerated bilharzial mass. The penile urethra is the commonest site of bilharziasis of the urethra. The ultimate result of bilharzial involvement of the urethra is fistula formation, or stricture of urethra.

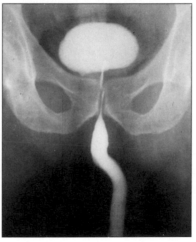

537 Bilharzial stricture of the posterior urethra. Note the elevated bladder base secondary to bilharzial bladder neck obstruction.

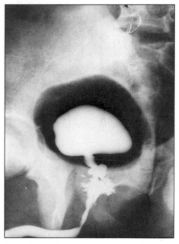

538 Urethral stricture with involvement of the prostate. Note again the raised and contracted bladder neck.

Bilharziasis of the seminal vesicles

539

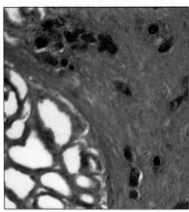

540

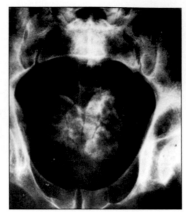

539 Section of a bilharzial seminal vesicle with multiple bilharzial ova. Note that the acini are not affected. The pathology starts in the fibromuscular part of the seminal vesicle and may remain as a closed lesion or it may extend to the mucous membrane of the acini causing ulceration and secondary infection, ending in fibrosis.

540 Plain radiograph showing the honey-comb appearance of calcified bilharzial seminal vesicle.

Bilharziasis of the prostate

541

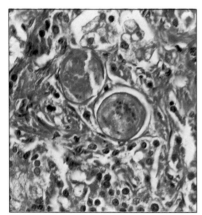

541 Bilharzial ova in the prostate. The disease commonly occurs on the vesical and urethral surface of the prostate because they are not covered by the thick capsule. Bilharzial nodules may occur in the para-prostatic plexus of veins and may be misdiagnosed as calculi, tubercle or malignant nodules. This section shows the ova in a prostate with adenocarcinoma. *(H&E × 256)*

6 Urinary tract stones

Over the last century, the process of Western industrialisation has resulted in a transition from the endemic bladder stone afflicting the young male child in economically poor countries to the idiopathic, predominantly calcium oxalate calculus of the affluent and developed nations. Approximately 70% of calculi in developed countries are composed of calcium oxalate with or without calcium phosphate. The prevalence of the idiopathic calcium-rich stone in the UK is approximately 3%, whereas in the USA 12% of males may ultimately form calculi. Stone disease in developed countries is considerably more common in males, and in 70–80% there is no obvious anatomical or biochemical cause. Urinary tract infection is responsible for 15–20% of stones occurring mainly in women, and inherited renal tubular syndromes and enzyme disorders account for only about 1% of stone formers. More than 50% of stone formers have recurrent episodes of stone formation.

Presenting symptoms

Patients with renal or ureteric calculi may present with loin pain, an attack of ureteric colic, haematuria, urinary tract infection, or less specific systemic symptoms as a result of sepsis. In addition stones in the lower ureter may occasionally present with an abrupt change in micturition.

Table 1 Pathogenesis of urinary calculi.

Type of disorder	Disorder
Idiopathic calcium stone disease	
Nonmetabolic disorders	Urinary tract infection
	Urinary diversion
	Congenital and obstructive disorders of the urinary tract
	Low urine output and dehydration (hot climate, diarrhoea, ileostomy)
	Foreign body
Metabolic disorders	
Hypercalciuria with hypercalcaemia	Primary hyperparathyroidism
	Idiopathic hypercalcaemia of infancy
	Milk–alkali syndrome
	Paget's disease of bone
Hypercalciuria with normocalcaemia	Idiopathic hypercalciuria (renal, absorptive)
	Medullary sponge kidney
	Renal tubular acidosis
Hypercalciuria with normocalcaemia or hypercalcaemia	Vitamin D intoxication
	Acute immobilisation
	Sarcoidosis
	Hyperthyroidism
	Cushing's disease
	Steroid therapy
	Malignancy
	Myelomatosis
Idiopathic hyperuricosuria	
Hyperuricaemic uric acid lithiasis	Gout
	Myeloproliferative disorders
	Lesch-Nyhan syndrome
Primary hyperoxaluria	
Secondary hyperoxaluria	Small bowel resection
	Crohn's disease
	Chronic pancreatitis
	Pancreatectomy
	Blind loop syndrome
	Tropical sprue
Cystinuria	
Xanthinuria	2,8 dihydroxyadenuria

Diagnostic investigations

The cornerstone of the diagnostic investigation is an IVU. Ultrasound or CT scanning may be useful in the diagnosis of radiolucent calculi or in defining the exact spatial anatomy in the planning of percutaneous surgery. Urine culture and renal function tests are essential investigations. Differential renal functions and creatinine clearance can be valuable when dealing with complex bilateral stone disease.

Table 2 Investigations to evaluate a stone former.

Type of test	Test
Radiology	IVU
Urine tests	Urine culture
	Urine microscopy for crystalluria
Metabolic investigations	
Urine	Volume
	pH
	Cystine spot test
24-hour urine collections	Calcium
	Uric acid
	Oxalate
	Citrate
Blood tests	Urea and electrolytes
	Creatinine
	Calcium
	Phosphate
	Uric acid
	Alkaline phosphatase
	Plasma proteins
	Chloride
	Bicarbonate
Chemical analysis of any stones formed	

Stone analysis

Quantitative chemical analysis of stones provides valuable information about their aetiology and may aid treatment. Although urinary calculi differ markedly in chemical and crystalline composition they all possess a common mucoprotein matrix core, consisting of protein and carbohydrate elements. This organic matrix scaffold for mineralisation tends to be arranged in concentric laminations with radical striations, but only contributes some 2.5–3.0% by weight. Cystine calculi may be composed of approximately 10% matrix, while the proportion of mucoprotein in the so-called pure matrix stone may reach 65%.

Accurate stone composition of very small stone fragments can be obtained using infra-red spectroscopy. Recent innovations with scanning electron microscopy combined with X-ray energy dispersive spectroscopy allow morphology and elemental analysis of stones to be correlated. Furthermore it is now becoming possible to forecast stone type from microanalysis of crystals within the urine of a stone former using similar techniques. This information can be used to predict the efficacy of stone disintegration.

Stone formation in cystinuria and hyperuricosuria results from excessive levels of cystine and uric acid respectively, with a low urinary pH contributing significantly to the latter.

Table 3 Stone types and their frequency.

Stone type	Approximate percentage of all stones
Calcium oxalate	26
Calcium oxalate and calcium phosphate	38
Calcium phosphates	7
Magnesium ammonium phosphate	20
Uric acid	6
Cystine	2

During the last decade, treatment of upper urinary tract calculi has undergone a revolution with the advent of extracorporeal shockwave lithotripsy, percutaneous renal surgery, and ureteroscopy in conjunction with various stone disintegrative techniques such as electrohydraulic lithotripsy, lasertripsy, ultrasonic lithotripsy and ballistic lithotripsy. Success depends on the ability to fragment calculi and hence stone fragility and its prediction has become an important consideration.

Examples of stones

542

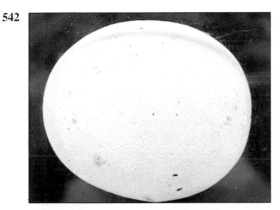

542 Phosphate stone. This is regular, spherical, and almost white.

543

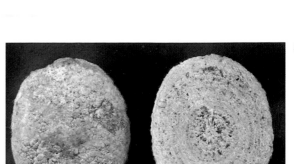

543 Phosphate stone. The surface is irregular and pitted, but on section laminations are clearly seen with the central areas.

544

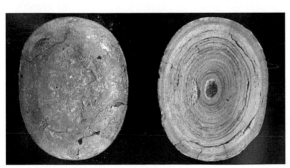

544 Uric acid stone. They show a brown discoloration caused by blood pigment. The stones are softer and the laminations and central nucleus are clearly seen. They are frequently radiolucent.

545

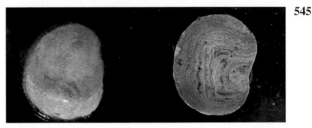

545 Uric acid stone. Another view, showing a more irregular stone in which the core is close to the periphery, probably caused by the splitting of the calculus.

546

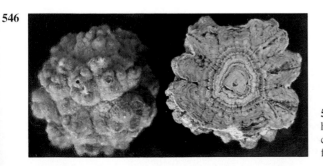

547

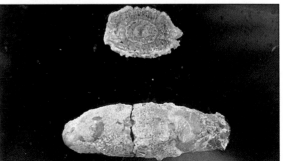

546, 547 Two examples of oxalate stone. They consist of mono-hydrate centres with secondary sharp spicules of the dihydrate crystals on the surface. Deposition of calcium phosphates will facilitate the development of a 'jackstone'.

129

Table 4 Stone composition.

Stone composition	Mineralogical name	Colour	Appearance	Stone fragility	Radiological density
Oxalates					
Calcium oxalate monohydrate	Whewellite	Dark brown to black	Dense and smooth	Intermediate fragmentation	Reasonably opaque
Calcium oxalate dihydrate	Weddellite	Yellow to light brown	Reticulated with scalloped edge	Total fragmentation	Reasonably opaque
Phosphates					
Calcium hydroxy-phosphate	Hydroxyapatite	Phosphates are highly variable in colour from pure white to off white through to yellow and dirty brown	Phosphates are usually hard, smooth with an irregular pitted surface, and often laminated	Intermediate fragmentation	Very opaque
Carbonate apatite	Carbonate apatite			Intermediate fragmentation	Very opaque
Calcium hydrogen phosphate dihydrate	Brushite			Poor fragmentation	Very opaque
Infective phosphates					
Magnesium ammonium phosphate hexahydrate	Struvite	Yellow-white	Smooth, soft and friable, grows rapidly into a staghorn configuration	Intermediate fragmentation	Slightly opaque
Uric acid and urates					
Uric acid		Yellow to reddish brown	Smooth, hard, with concentric laminations	Total fragmentation	Radiolucent if pure
Ammonium acid Urate Sodium acid urate monohydrate		Yellow	Soft and friable	Total fragmentation	Radiolucent if pure
Others					
Cystine	Cystine S	Opaque yellow-blue	Smooth, glistening and waxy	Very poor fragmentation	Slightly opaque
	Cystine R	Dark tan resembling honey	Rough crystalline surface	Intermediate fragmentation	Slightly opaque
Xanthine		Yellow-brown	Smooth and soft		Radiolucent

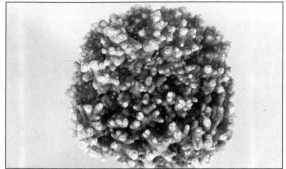

548 Mulberry stone, mostly oxalate.

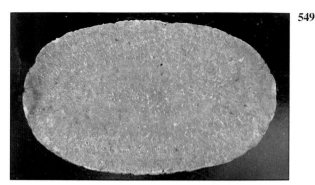

549 Cystine stone. The stone is blue in colour, interspaced with white areas caused by a combination of amino acids. The finding of cystine on urine screening must always be followed by an examination of a 24-hour specimen for all amino acids by amino acid chromatography in affected patients; the worst cases are in the homozygous group. The stones may be radio-lucent. Because cystine is the most insoluble, there is a tree-like appearance with a very irregular surface and shape. The elongated shape is typical of a stone shaped to the pattern of a ureter.

Further examples of calculi

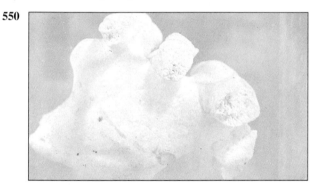

550 Staghorn calculus (usually phosphate).

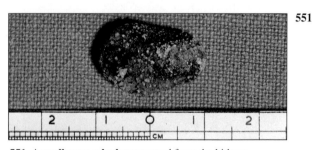

551 A mulberry calculus removed from the kidney.

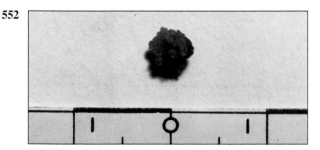

552 An irregular-shaped calculus removed from the ureter.

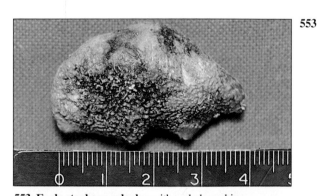

553 Early staghorn calculus with early branching.

Hyperparathyroidism

'Bones, stones, moans, and abdominal groans'

Patients with hyperparathyroidism account for 4–12% of stone formers. Primary hyperparathyroidism occurs in approximately 0.1% of the population, with 45% presenting with urinary tract stones. The combination of persistent hypercalcaemia and a low serum phosphate is highly suggestive of hyperparathyroidism and assays for parathormone are now widely available to confirm the diagnosis. Biochemical screening has gone a long way to identifying patients with subtle or intermittent hyperparathyroidism, but in some cases a provocative oral calcium challenge is necessary to establish the diagnosis.

Hyperparathyroidism can result from parathyroid tumours, either single or multiple, parathyroid hyperplasia, or rarely parathyroid calciuria, all of which produce an excess of parathormone. Diagnosis must be established biochemically, but pre-surgical localisation can be performed with technetium and thallium subtraction scanning, which localise approximately 80% of parathyroid adenomas and are particularly important with recurrent disease.

The high serum calcium occurs as a result of mobilisation of calcium from the bone because of the increased activity of the osteoclasts. This osteoclasis causes changes in the bone, which may be the sole manifestation of the hyperparathyroidism, but may also be associated with renal calculi or calcification in other areas of the body. The first change that may occur is a diffuse osteoclasis, which results in generalised osteoporosis.

554

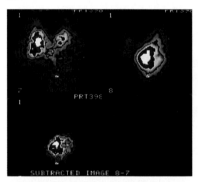

554 Technetium and thallium subtraction scan demonstrating a parathyroid adenoma with the subtracted image.

555

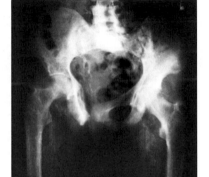

555 Generalised osteoporosis produces lack of mineralisation in the bone; the basketwork appearance is shown in the femur.

556

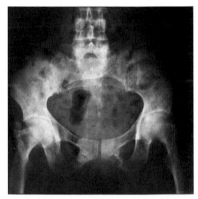

556 Pathological fracture resulting from demineralisation in the neck of the femur. Localised cystic areas may occur. They can be either multiple or single.

557

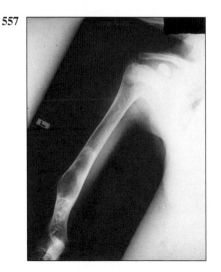

557 A cyst in the humerus. These cysts may have a thin sclerotic margin. On the other hand they may show no evidence of dense surrounding bone. Fractures in this type of lesion are common. Localised subperiosteal lesions are diagnostic of hyperparathyroidism. They are seen in the phalanges and are again caused by osteoclasis.

558 A subperiosteal lesion. This may present as one or two small pits in the cortex of the phalanges of a finger or multiple pits, which produce an irregular edge deep to the periosteum. The latest stage is a lace-like pattern as seen; this is caused by the laying down of new subperiosteal bone. Hyperparathyroidism can also cause calcification in other systems.

558

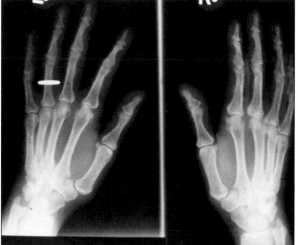

559

560

559 Diffuse calcification in peripheral vessels.

560 Calcification in the pancreas combined with a staghorn calculus in a diabetic patient.

561

562

Calcification in other sites in the upper abdomen can sometimes lead to difficulties in diagnosis on plain films.

561 Ring shadow of splenic artery calcification.

562 Diffuse pancreatic calcification.

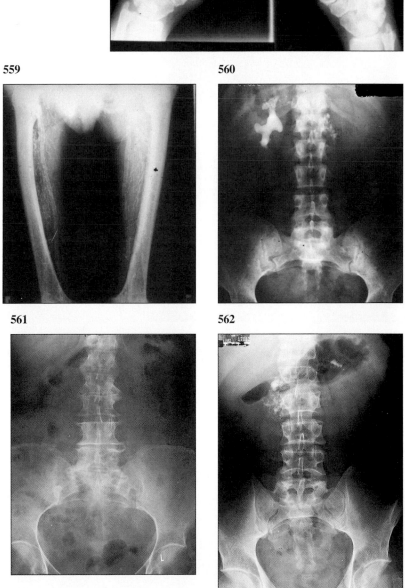

133

Renal calculi

563

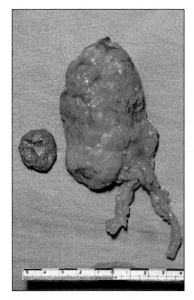

564

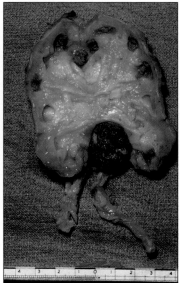

Untreated stone disease can lead to complete renal destruction.

563, 564 Two examples of damage caused by untreated calculi. This calculus obstructed the pelviureteric junction completely destroying the kidney, which is shrunken and scarred with gross cortical destruction and with calculi in dilated calyces.

Patients with congenital abnormalities are particularly prone to stone disease especially if the abnormalities lead to stasis.

565

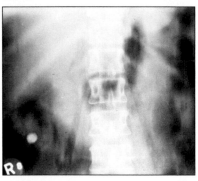

566

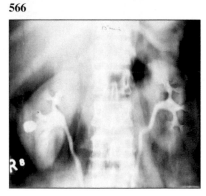

565, 566 Straight KUB* and IVU showing large calyceal calculus producing minimal renal damage. This is a stone within a calyceal cyst.

567

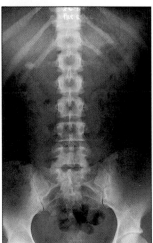

568

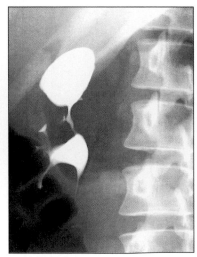

567, 568 KUB and right ureterogram of stasis stone in calyceal diverticulum. Ureterography elegantly demonstrates this calyceal diverticulum and its retained stone with the connection to the calyceal system.

* A KUB is a plain straight abdominal radiograph showing kidneys, ureters, and bladder.

569, 570 Calculi can occupy the whole of one moiety of a duplex system. KUB and IVU.

569

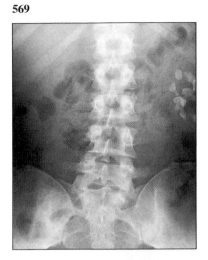

570

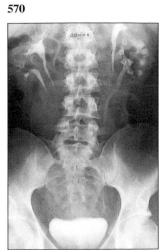

571, 572 KUB and IVU of a calyceal stone within the middle moiety of a triplex system.

571

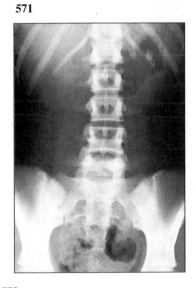

572

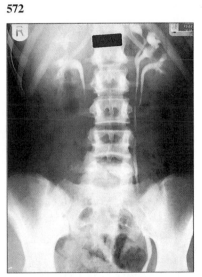

573, 574 KUB and IVU of stone in upper part of crossed renal ectopia.

573

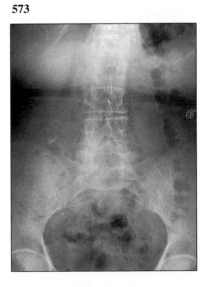

574

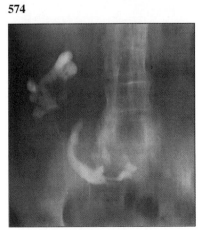

575

576

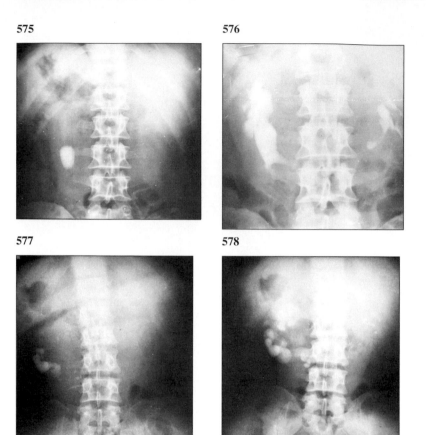

**575, 576 KUB and IVU of a horseshoe
kidney containing a single calculus** in
the right renal pelvis.

577

578

**577, 578 KUB and IVU of multiple
calculi** in the right pelvis of a horseshoe
kidney causing pelvicalyceal obstruction.

Pelviureteric junction (PUJ) obstruction
Stasis leads to multiple stones in the dilated collecting system.

579

580

581

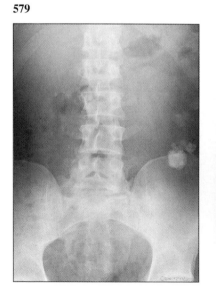

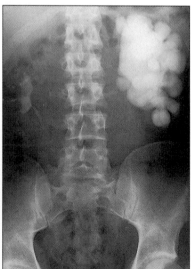

**581 Kidney destroyed by renal
calculus**, which has obstructed the pelviureteric junction. There is almost total
destruction, leaving only a thin shell of
renal tissue.

579, 580 KUB and IVU of congenital pelviureteric obstruction.

Megaureters

582, 583 KUB and IVU showing stones in both kidneys and in the grossly dilated lower left ureter.

Multiple renal stones may arise in relation to congenital defects as in medullary sponge kidney or metabolic problems such as renal tubular acidosis and nephrocalcinosis.

582

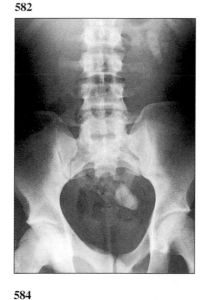

583

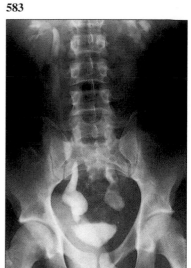

Medullary sponge kidney

Medullary sponge kidney is congenital and is usually diagnosed after 20 years of age, particularly in middle age. It is manifested as small cysts in relation to the pyramids, which appear as rounded cavities full of dye on IVU, may be unilateral or bilateral, and may or may not contain calculi. If calculi are present it is difficult to distinguish from nephrocalcinosis. About 30% of patients have idiopathic hypercalciuria.

584, 585 KUB and IVU of moderate degree of medullary sponge kidney.

584

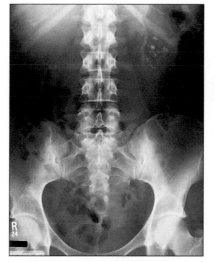

585

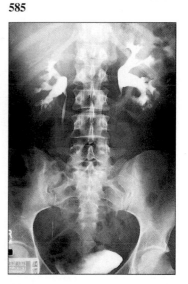

586, 587 Advanced medullary sponge kidney with calcification.

586

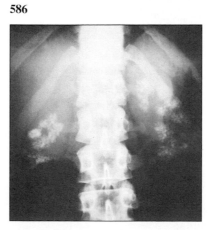

587

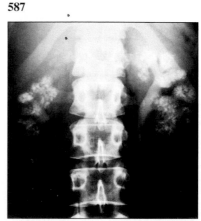

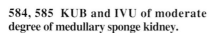

588

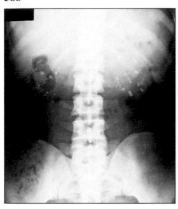

Renal tubular acidosis

Renal tubular acidosis is one of the causes of nephrocalcinosis. It is an inherited condition, transmitted by an autosomal recessive gene, which leads to failure to acidify the urine. The characteristic presentation is a low plasma bicarbonate accompanied by alkaline urine. The diagnosis is confirmed by failure of the urine to become acid 6 hours after a loading dose of ammonium chloride, 0.1 g/kg body weight over 1 hour. For this test to be accurate the urine must be sterile.

588 Renal tubular acidosis with calcification.

Nephrocalcinosis

Occasionally calcium is deposited in the substance of the kidney and is referred to as nephrocalcinosis. This can be macroscopic or microscopic. The principal causes are hyperparathyroidism, malignancy, myelomatosis, Paget's disease of bone, renal tubular acidosis, medullary sponge kidney, vitamin D intoxication, the milk–alkali syndrome, sarcoidosis, and idiopathic hypercalciuria. It may or may not be accompanied by renal calculi.

589

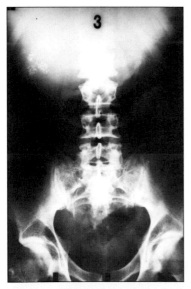

589 An example of early nephro-calcinosis.

590

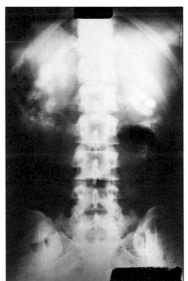

591

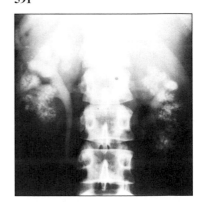

590, 591 KUB and IVU of severe nephrocalcinosis.

592

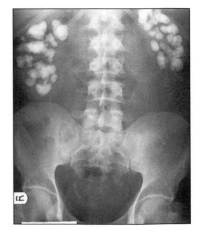

592 Very advanced nephrocalcinosis with spontaneous stone street.

Papillary necrosis

Calcification can also be seen in renal papillary necrosis. This is a late development and is due to calcification of necrotic papillae, which gives rise to a picture very similar to nephrocalcinosis. The commonest causes are diabetes, analgesic abuse, prolonged infection, and sickle-cell disease.

Stones may also arise as a result of other disease or operations.

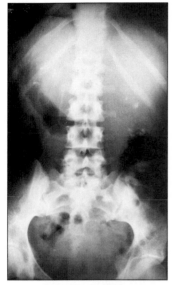
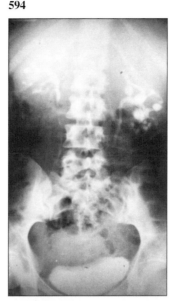

593, 594 KUB and IVU of an advanced degree of calcification in papillary necrosis secondary to diabetes.

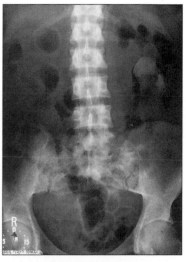

595 Following urinary diversion stones may arise in the upper tracts. Air pyelogram showing a partial left staghorn with peripheral stones on the right following an ileal conduit diversion.

Examples of calculi of different chemical composition

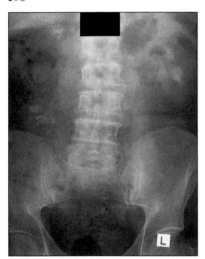
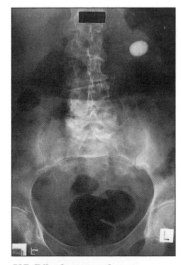
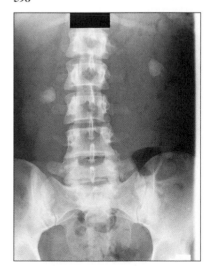

596 Struvite staghorn stone formation in a solitary left kidney.

597 Dihydrate renal stone.

598 Bilateral cystine stones. These sometimes show ring shadows.

599

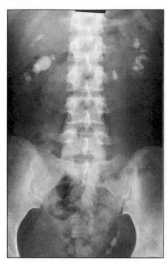

600

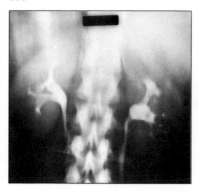

599 Primary hyperoxaluria. A 16-year-old girl with aggressive bilateral disease.

600 Uric acid calculi are not radio-opaque and are only diagnosed in the kidney when they produce a filling defect in the pelvis on an IVU. IVU showing a filling defect in the renal pelvis caused by a uric acid stone.

601

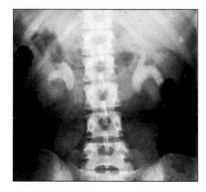

602

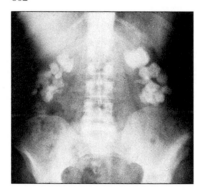

Staghorn calculi

601 Early staghorn calculus, which is beginning to branch.

602 Bilateral staghorn.

603

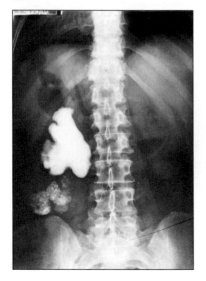

604

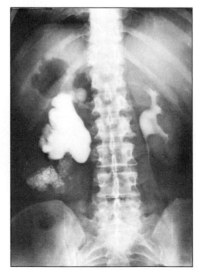

603, 604 KUB and IVU of a staghorn calculus with an additional group of calculi in the dilated lower pole calyx.

605

606

607

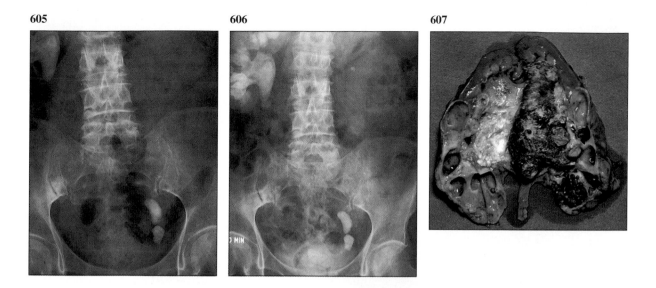

608

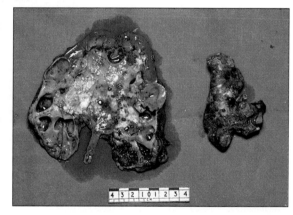

605, 606 KUB and IVU of right staghorn calculus with left lower ureteric stones and very poor function on that side. The right side has retained reasonable function.

607, 608 The effect of a staghorn calculus on the kidney, emphasising the seriousness of any neglected calculus.

609 Typical pigmented staghorn calculus. It was composed of calcium phosphate and magnesium ammonium phosphate.

610, 611 IVU and micturating cystogram showing staghorn calculus secondary to ureteric reflux. This investigation must always be carried out in patients with staghorn calculi.

609

610

611

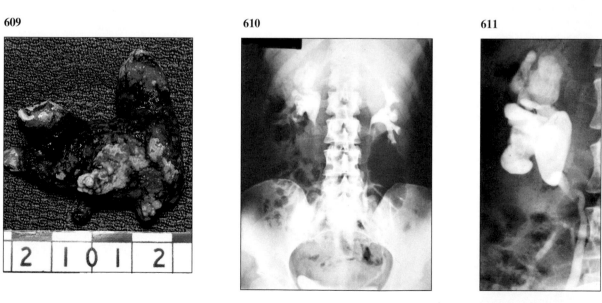

612

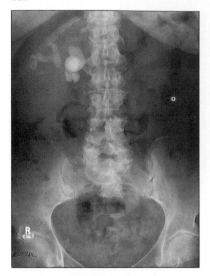

613

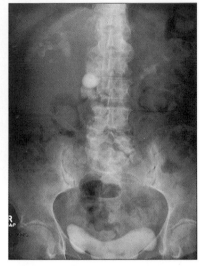

Complications of renal stones

Complications of staghorn calculi include total destruction and non-function of the affected kidney by infection and stones together with the development of a perinephric abscess.

612 Plain KUB film showing staghorn calculus together with calcification within an extrarenal abscess.

613 An IVU demonstrates normal function of the left kidney and no function of the affected right side.

614

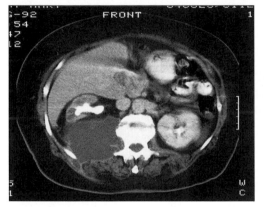

615

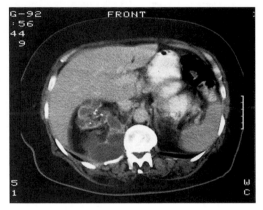

614 Staghorn calculus lying in the atrophic right kidney, a large abscess cavity posterior to the kidney, and a normal left kidney.

615 Intrarenal and upper ureteric sepsis together with a loculated cavity posteriorly.

616

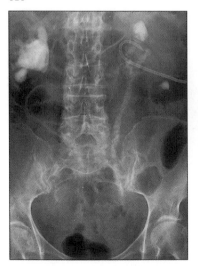

616 Bilateral staghorn calculi. Note the very extensive stone street (Steine Strasse) following extracorporeal shockwave lithotripsy (ESWL) therapy. Nephrostomy tube *in situ*.

617

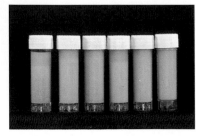

617 Very large volume of stone street passed in a single void.

Ureteric calculi

Renal calculi may become dislodged and cause ureteric obstruction, which produces ureteric colic; this will be the initial presenting symptom.

618

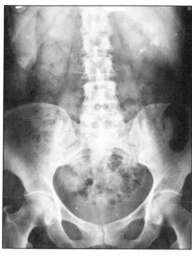

619

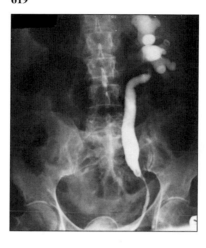

620

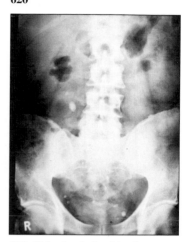

620 Calculus lodged in the upper third of the ureter.

618, 619 KUB and retrograde pyelogram in which part of a renal calculus has obstructed the ureter causing hydroureter and hydronephrosis. Ureteric calculi can obstruct in the upper, middle, or lower third of the ureter.

621

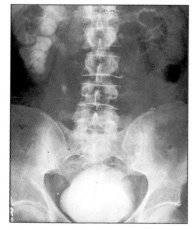

622

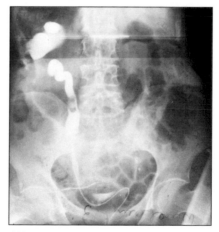

623

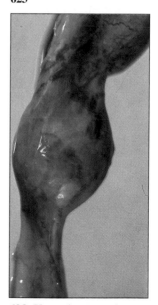

621 Calculus lodged in the middle third of the ureter.

622 Urate calculus, which is almost non-opaque to X-rays, obstructing the middle third of the ureter.

623 Ureteric stone. A post-mortem specimen of a ureter showing a bulge caused by a stone (in the centre of the field), a normal ureter below the bulge, and a dilated ureter above it.

624

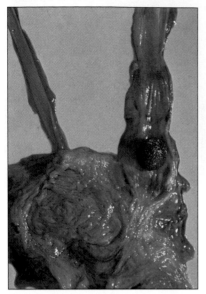

624 Ureteric stone. The previous specimen dissected to show a unilateral hydroureter caused by a stone a short distance above the bladder.

625

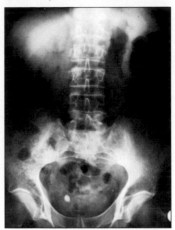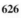

626

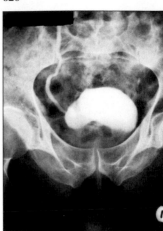

625, 626 KUB and IVU of calculus situated in the lower third of the ureter close to the ureterovesical junction.

Ureteroscopy

Ureteroscopy is extremely helpful in the diagnosis and management of renal pelvic and ureteric calculi.

627

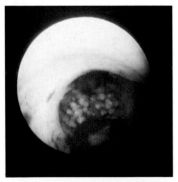

627 Ureteroscopy of calculus in renal pelvis.

628

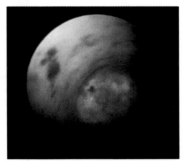

628 Ureteroscopy of calculus in ureter.

629

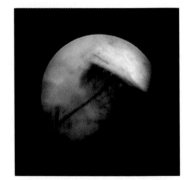

629 Ureteroscopy of calculus captured within Dormia basket.

630, 631, 632, 633 The effect of a calculus is unpredictable. Sometimes the same size of calculus causes obstruction as shown in **630** and **631**. On other occasions there is free ureteric drainage, as **632** and **633** demonstrate.

630

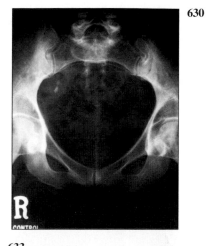

631

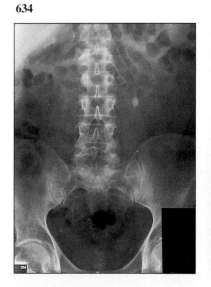

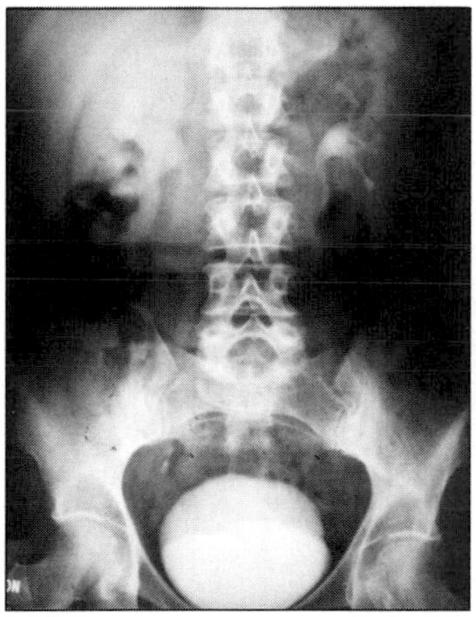

632

633

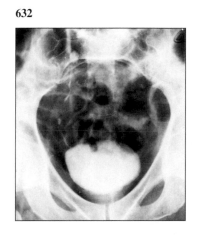

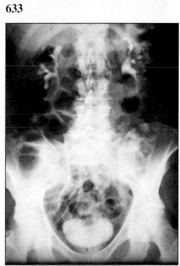

634, 635 Gross obstruction can follow impaction of a stone in the upper ureter. KUB and IVU.

634

635

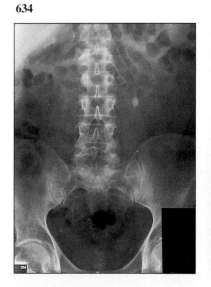

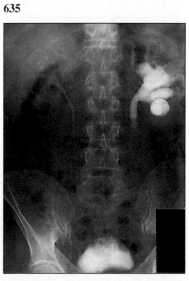

Ureteric calculi occasionally form in ureteroceles.

636

637

638

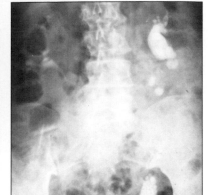

639

640

641

642

636, 637 Calculus in a ureterocele, which is at the lower end of the duplex system. The ureters join just above the ureterovesical junction.

638 Multiple calculi in a ureterocele, kidney, and ureter.

639 A large ureteric calculus, which passed spontaneously. Large ureteric calculi can occasionally pass through the intramural part of the ureter. Calculi of this size must however be watched carefully because they rarely pass spontaneously.

640 Dormia basket with engaged stone in lower third of ureter. Note stone street in upper ureter. Nephrostomy tube *in situ*.

641, 642 A calculus removed by a Dormia basket, a technique that can be used if the calculus is small and no ureteric dilatation is evident.

643 Dangers of using Dormia basket. The basket wires can break and may then become detached.

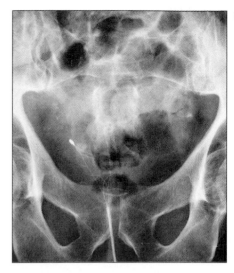

Investigation of ureteric obstruction

644 A dense nephrogram following injection of intravenous contrast medium shows the classical appearance in an acutely obstructed kidney. This investigation has hazards in the grossly obstructed system.

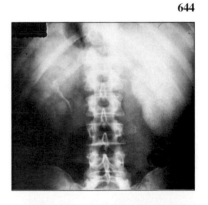

645 Plain film.

646 After contrast. A nephrostogram reveals gross obstruction produced by the lower ureteric stone and allows drainage of the upper tract.

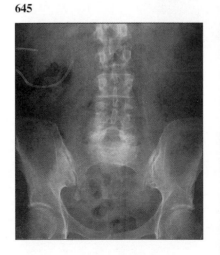

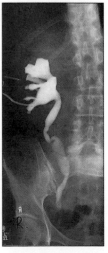

647

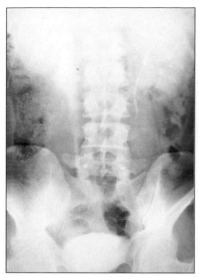

648

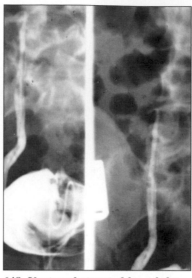

649

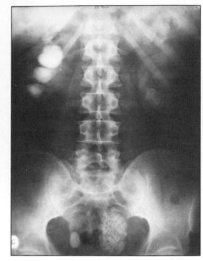

647 IVU showing spontaneous rupture in an acutely obstructed upper urinary tract. The ureteric obstruction seen here is due to sulphonamide crystal formation and is rarely found today.

648 Ureter obstructed by sulphon-amide crystals. Note the linear pattern and the filling defect in the bladder, which is caused by blood clot.

649 KUB of calculi in the kidney, ureter, and a bladder diverticulum. On rare occasions calculi can involve multiple parts of the renal tract.

Ureteric stents

Ureteric stents have revolutionised the management of stone disease by lithotripsy. Stones can, however, form in relation to stents.

650

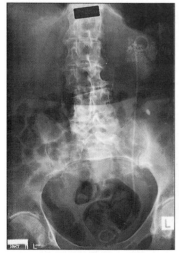

651

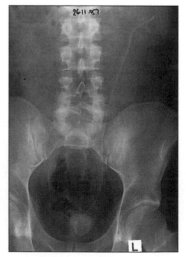

652

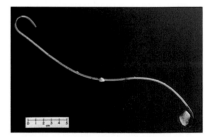

652 Stent removed with stones attached.

650 Double pigtail stent in left ureter.

651 Stones can form on a stent.

653 Stents can fragment when left long term.

654 Stents do prevent the formation of gross stone streets, as seen here filling the whole ureter.

653

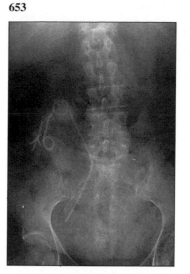

654

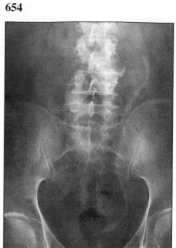

Bladder calculi

Bladder calculi may be primary or secondary. Primary calculi are rare in Western countries, but are common in India, Pakistan, Iran, Egypt, and other Middle-eastern countries. Secondary calculi may form around a stone that has come from the kidney, but are much more likely to result from bladder outlet obstruction. Calculi rarely form over a foreign body, which acts as a nucleus.

Bladder calculi vary in size, colour, shape, and number and their composition is similar to renal stones. Small stones must be distinguished from phleboliths, which are calcification in pelvic veins, are usually numerous, and are situated outside the line of the ureter and lateral to the bladder outline. Ultrasound is less effective than radiology in the assessment of stone disease.

655

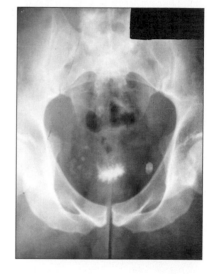

655 Phleboliths.

656 Ultrasound of a large intravesical calculus reveals the classical back shadow projected by the calculus onto the surrounding tissue. This can be compared with the intravesical image formed by a similar sized bladder tumour (see p. 207, **927**).

657 Small bladder stone.

658 Larger bladder stone.

656

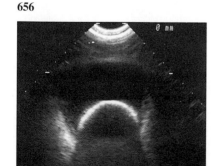

657

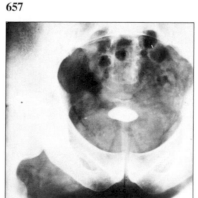

658

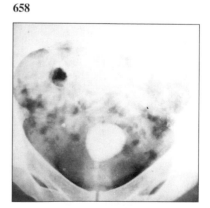

659

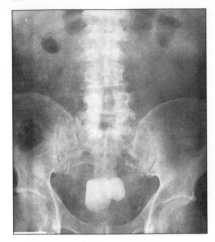

660

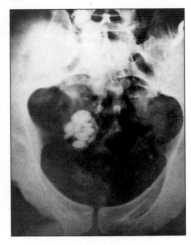

659 Multiple bladder stones.

660 Multiple bladder stones in a bladder diverticulum.

661

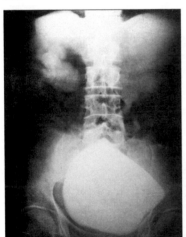

661, 662, 663 Large bladder stone. This stone was removed by one of the authors and weighed 2.1 kg. The patient ultimately died of squamous cell carcinoma of the bladder.

662

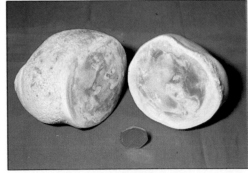

663

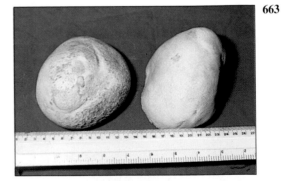

664

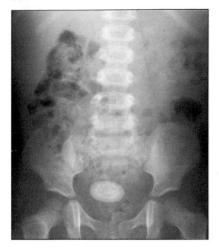

665

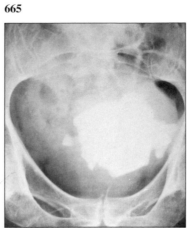

666

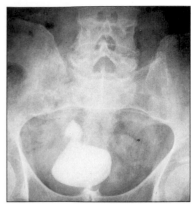

664 Large bladder stone in an Asian child. These are seen in children, particularly in the Indian subcontinent and around the Pacific rim and are of dietary origin.

667

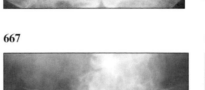
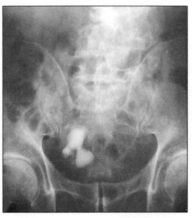

668

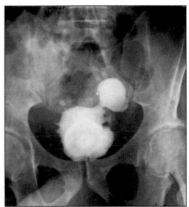

Calculi of unusual shape

665 Large calculus with a very irregular surface.

666 Single calculus in a diverticulum, which has the appearance of a ring shadow.

667 Dumbell appearance.

668 Large calculus involving the bladder and a diverticulum.

669, 670 Large calculus causing varying degrees of obstruction to the upper urinary tract.

669

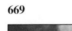
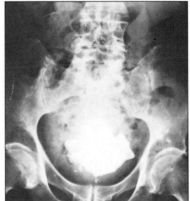

670

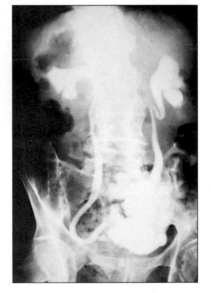

671

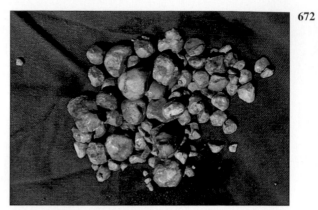

672

672 **Multiple mixed stones** removed during a prostatectomy.

671 **Mulberry calculus** removed from the bladder. It is identical to the renal mulberry stone.

Endoscopic appearances of calculi

673

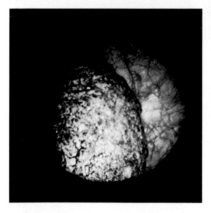

674

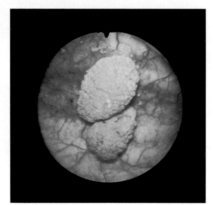

673 **Mulberry stone with mild degree of cystitis**.

674 **Two irregular rough calculi**.

675 Outflow obstruction causing numerous small calculi. Note the trabeculation.

676 A calculus with severe cystitis.

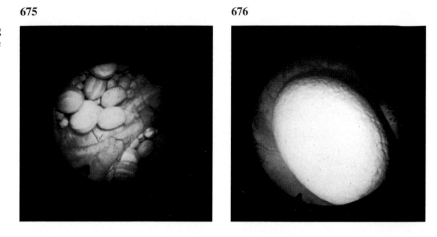

677 A calculus with a minor degree of inflammation.

678 A soft stone combined with severe infection.

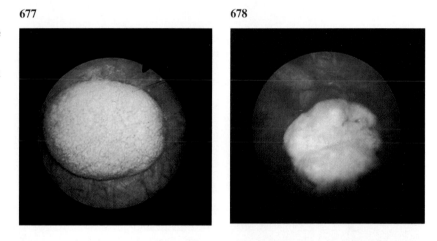

679 Multiple small calculi secondary to bladder outlet obstruction.

680 Endoscopic view of jackstone in the bladder.

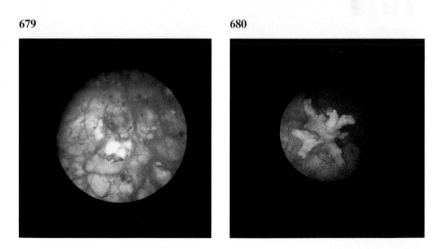

681

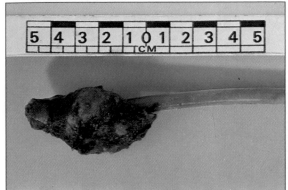

681 Bladder stone. A calculus forming on the tip of a catheter, which had been left in the bladder for a long time.

682

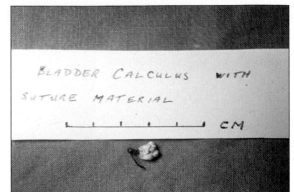

682 Calculi occasionally form over a foreign body. Bladder calculus formed over nonabsorbable suture material, which had inadvertently included the bladder during pelvic surgery.

683

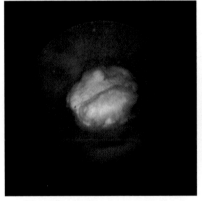

683 Larger bladder calculus formed over suture material. The calculus remained securely attached to the bladder wall. Part of the bladder had to be resected.

684

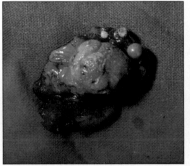

684 Calcification involves the whole of the thickness of the bladder wall.

685

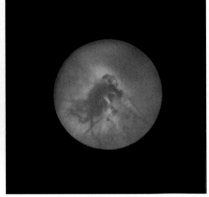

685 A rare cause of bladder calculi is irradiation cystitis. An area of irradiation cystitis on which small calculi have formed. They are usually pigmented and are basically composed of calcium oxalate.

686

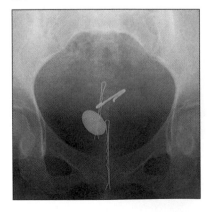

686 Foreign bodies of many types have been reported in the bladder and most of these have been introduced along anatomical channels. Among many described are pieces of endoscopic instruments, a urethral catheter coated with phosphatic secretion, slippery elm bark, hair pins, safety pins, pencils, wire, and paper clips. These are but a few of an almost end-less number of bizarre articles.

687

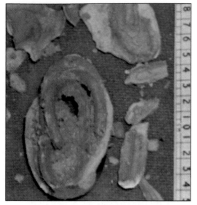

688

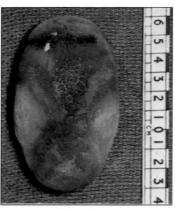

689

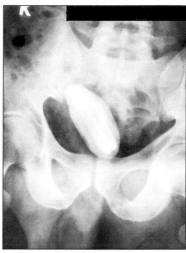

687 Calcified catheter removed from the bladder.

688 Same foreign body before destruction.

689 Urogram of same foreign body.

Calcification occurs in the prostate and can be associated with bladder outlet obstruction. It is always multiple and may take the form of multiple prostatic calculi.

690

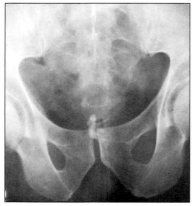

691

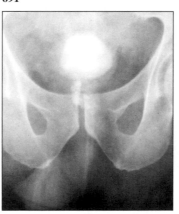

692

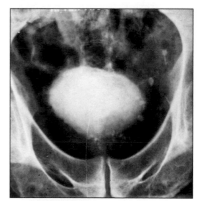

690, 691 KUB and IVU showing prostatic calcification associated with early bladder outlet obstruction.

692 IVU showing prostatic calcification associated with gross bladder outlet obstruction and trabeculation; note the numerous phleboliths.

155

693

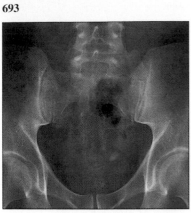

694

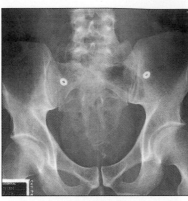

695

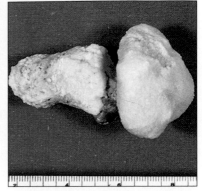

693, 694 Left ureteric calculus which has moved down spontaneously into prostatic urethra.

695 Calculus removed from prostate. Note the waist in the middle because part of the calculus was in the bladder and part was in the prostatic urethra.

Urethral calculi

696

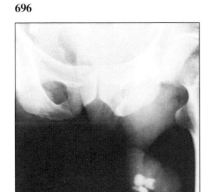

697

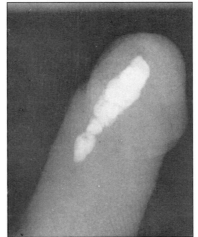

Calculi are occasionally found in the urethra. They are always secondary to bladder calculi unless they form in a urethral diverticulum. They usually come to light when they wedge in the urethra and cause urinary obstruction.

696 Calculi in a urethral diverticulum.

697 Spindle-shaped calculus impacted in the penile urethra.

698

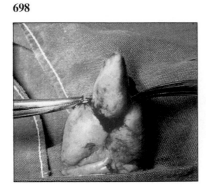

699

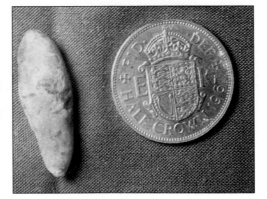

698, 699 Calculus presenting at the urethral orifice and after extraction.

7 Disorders of the kidney and ureter

Renal tumours

Patients with tumours of the renal substance, renal pelvis, or ureter most commonly present with haematuria. They may also complain of loin pain. A loin mass may be present as a result of either the renal tumour itself, or as a result of hydronephrosis produced by ureteric obstruction.

Unusual presentations include haematological disturbances such as polycythaemia, pyrexia of unknown origin (PUO), and symptoms from metastatic deposits usually in the bones or in the chest.

Most of the tumours encountered in clinical practice are renal cortical carcinomas, nephroblastomas, or transitional cell carcinomas. The other primary tumours are much less common. It is rare for a metastasis to present in the kidney, but at autopsy secondary deposits in the kidney are not uncommon.

Tumours of the kidney

- Renal cortical carcinoma (hypernephroma, renal adenocarcinoma, Grawitz tumour, renal carcinoma).
- Oncocytoma.
- Nephroblastoma (Wilms' tumour).
- Connective tissue tumours (e.g. leiomyoma).
- Tumour-like lesions (e.g. hamartoma, solitary cyst).

Tumours of the renal pelvis and ureter

- Epithelial tumours (carcinoma).
- Connective tissue tumours.
- Tumour-like lesions (e.g. fibroepithelial polyp, malakoplakia).

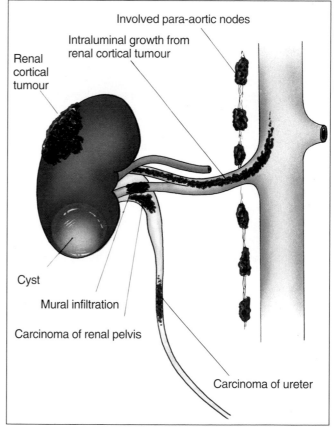

700

700 Schematic representation of tumours of the kidney, pelvis, and ureter. Calcification is found in some renal tumours.

Renal cortical tumours—TNM clinical classification*

Minimum requirements for assessment

- **T** Clinical examination, urography, and arteriography before definitive treatment.
- **N** Clinical examination and radiography, including lymphography and urography. Venocavography is recommended.
- **M** Clinical examination and radiography.

T (primary tumour)

TX Primary tumour cannot be assessed.
T0 No evidence of primary tumour.
T1 Tumour 2.5 cm or less in greatest dimension.
T2 Tumour more than 2.5 cm in greatest dimension, but limited to kidney.

T3 Tumour extends into major veins or invades adrenal gland or perinephric tissues, but not beyond Gerota's fascia.

    T3a Tumour invades adrenal gland or perinephric tissues, but not beyond Gerota's fascia.

    T3b Tumour grossly extends into the renal vein(s) or vena cava below the diaphragm.

    T3c Tumour grossly extends into the vena cava above the diaphragm.

T4 Tumour invades beyond Gerota's fascia.

N (regional and juxtaregional lymph nodes)

The regional lymph nodes are the para-aortic nodes and the paracaval nodes. The juxtaregional lymph nodes are the intrapelvic nodes and the supraclavicular nodes.

N0 No evidence of regional lymph node involvement.
N1 Evidence of involvement of a single homolateral regional lymph node.
N2 Evidence of involvement of contralateral or bilateral or multiple regional lymph nodes.

N3 Evidence of involvement of juxtaregional lymph nodes (assessable only at surgical exploration).
N4 Evidence of involvement of juxtaregional lymph nodes.
NX The minimum requirements to assess the regional and/or juxtaregional lymph nodes cannot be met.

M (distant metastases)

M0 No evidence of distant metastases.
M1 Evidence of distant metastases (specify, using recommended abbreviations).

MX The minimum requirements to assess the regional and/or juxtaregional lymph nodes cannot be met.

Further postsurgical histopathological classification (pTNM)

- **pT** (primary tumour) categories corresponding to the T categories.
- **pN** (regional and juxtaregional lymph nodes) categories correspond to the N categories.
- **pM** (distant metastases) categories correspond to the M categories.
- **Invasion of veins** (V): **V0**, veins do not contain tumour; **V1** renal vein contains tumour; **V2**, vena cava contains tumour; **VX**, venous invasion cannot be assessed.
- **Histopathological grading (G)**: **G1**, high degree of differentiation; **G2**, medium; **G3**, low or undifferentiated; **GX**, not assessed.
- **Additional descriptions**: prefix **r** for recurrent cases; prefix **y** for cases having other treatment before surgery.

* Adapted from *TNM Classification of Malignant Tumours* 4th edition, 2nd revision. 1992, Springer Verlag.

Stage grouping (Robson 1969)

There are four stages in the Robson system:

- **Stage I** Tumour is confined to the kidney.
- **Stage II** Tumour extends through the renal capsule and invades the perinephric fat, but is contained within the renal fascia (Gerota's fascia).
- **Stage III** Tumour has invaded the renal vein or the regional lymph nodes or both, with or without involvement of the vena cava or perinephric fat.
- **Stage IV** Tumour has metastasised to distant sites (including distant lymph nodes) or has extended through the renal fascia to involve contiguous structures.

Nephroblastoma—pretreatment clinical classification (TNM)

T (primary tumour)

TX Primary tumour cannot be assessed.
T0 No evidence of primary tumour.
T1 Evidence of unilateral tumour 80 cm^2 or less in area (including kidney).
T2 Evidence of unilateral tumour more than 80 cm^2 in area (including kidney) (Note: the area is calculated by multiplying the vertical and horizontal dimensions of the radiological shadow of the tumour and kidney).

T3 Evidence of unilateral tumour rupture before treatment.
T4 Evidence of bilateral tumours before treatment.
TX The minimum requirements to assess the primary tumour cannot be met.

N (regional lymph nodes)

The regional lymph nodes are the hilar nodes, the para-aortic nodes, and the paracaval nodes between the diaphragm and the bifurcation of the aorta. Other involved lymph nodes are considered as distant metastases.
N0 No evidence of lymph node involvement.

N1 Evidence of regional lymph node involvement.
NX The minimum requirements to assess the regional lymph nodes cannot be met.

M (distant metastases)

M0 No evidence of distant metastases.
M1 Evidence of distant metastases.

MX The minimum requirements to assess the presence of distant metastases cannot be met.

Further postsurgical histopathological classification (TNM)
This can be added as with renal cortical tumours.

Clinical stage grouping (TNM)

- Stage I: T1; N0, NX; M0.
- Stage II: T2; N0, NX; M0.
- Stage III: T1, T2; N1; M0 or T3; any N; M0.

- Stage IV: T1, T2, T3; any N; M1.
- Stage V: T4; any N; any M.

701

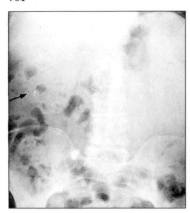

702

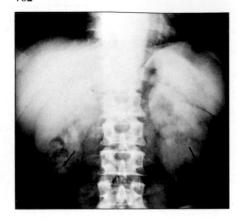

Plain radiography of the abdomen

The renal outlines can be seen and the enlargement of the contour of the right lower pole indicates a space-occupying lesion, in this case a tumour.

701 Diffuse stippling in a right renal tumour.

702 Peripheral tumours may be defined with tomography.

Intravenous urography (IVU)

Intravenous urography (IVU) is still an invaluable investigation in patients suspected of having a renal tumour.

703

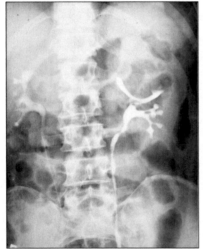

704

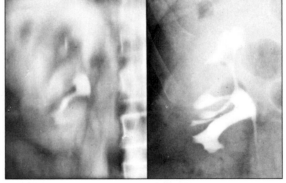

703 Calyceal distortion with stretching and separation of the calyces indicates a space-occupying lesion.

704 Calyceal destruction indicates tumour invasion of the drainage system.

705 The renal pelvis can also be invaded.

705

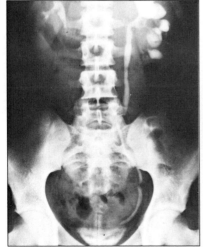

Ureterography

706

707

706, 707 The technique of ascending contrast studies is invaluable in demonstrating destruction of the pelvicalyceal system in nonfunctioning kidneys, due to malignant disease.

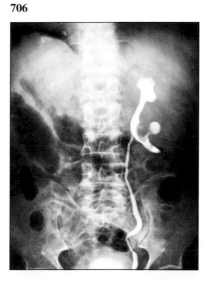

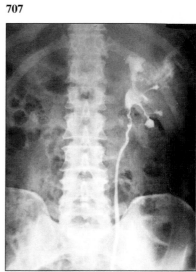

Renal arteriography

This study shows both kidneys by the flood technique or individual systems by selective arteriograms.

708 Flood films show the vascular pattern of both kidneys. Right normal, left distorted by malignant disease.

709 The late phase shows the normal right kidney and the enlarged left kidney showing diffuse tumour circulation.

708

709

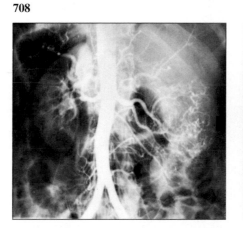

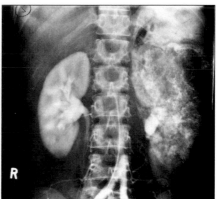

710

711

712

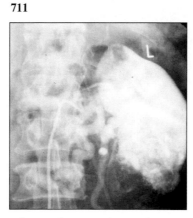

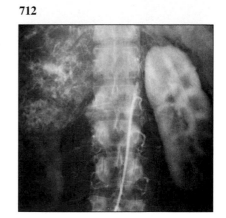

710, 711 Early and late selective films show the vascular pattern in a renal tumour.

712 An example of the early phase shows the normal dense left nephrogram with the 'tumour blush' of fine pathological vessels on the contralateral side.

713

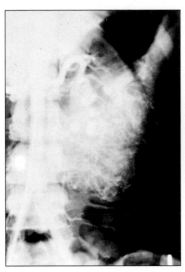

714

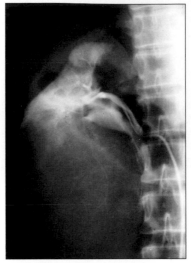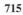

715

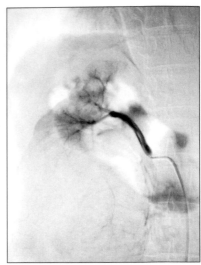

713 Selective film showing arterio-venous fistulas in a large tumour. There is laking or pooling of contrast medium.

714, 715 Subtraction films may be helpful. An arteriogram and subtraction arteriogram are shown here.

716

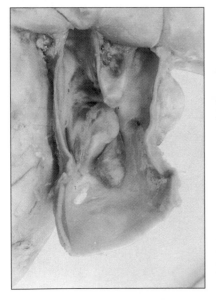

717

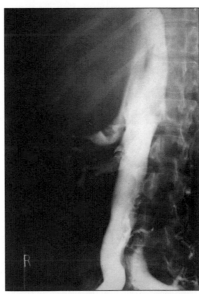

Vascular invasion

Renal cortical tumours may spread, with extension of the tumour within the lumen of the renal vein and cava, and it may invade the walls of these vessels.

716 Dissection of the main renal vein of a formalin-fixed specimen with elevations on the inner wall of the vein where the tumour in the kidney is growing through into the vein.

Cavography

717 Tumour visible in renal vein.

718

719

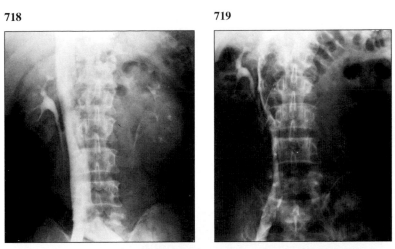

718, 719 Early and late involvement of the cava. See also **759** and **760**, p.171.

Ultrasound

This technique will show whether a space-occupying lesion is solid or cystic by the presence or absence of 'echoes'.

720, 721 Ultrasound studies, longitudinal (**720**) and transverse (**721**), show distortion of the renal outline by a superficial echogenic mass suggesting a solid renal tumour.

720

721

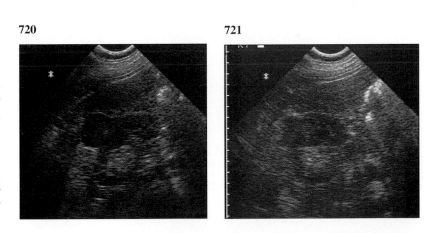

722 A CT study in the same patient as that shown in 720 and 721 after contrast shows partial enhancement of a mass lesion on the lateral surface of right kidney.

722

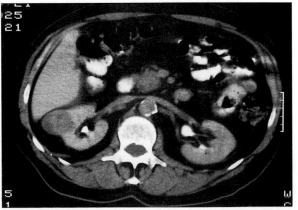

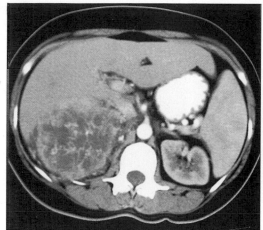

CT scanning

Computerised axial tomography of the renal image shows the variation of density exhibited by the renal tumour on transverse abdominal 'cuts' and will also indicate gland masses when present.

723 A large renal tumour appearing as a partly solid mass with classical areas of necrosis within it.

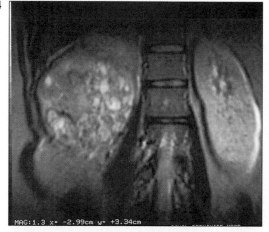

MRI scanning

CT with contrast is the first-line approach to the investigation of renal cortical carcinomas, but MRI tends to be used for problem cases where the multiplanar facilities will answer specific questions.

724, 725, 726 The same tumour as in 723 is seen in **724**, occupying the whole of the upper pole of the right kidney. MRI is also very useful for detecting involvement of other organs. The CT scan (**725**) suggests that there is liver involvement by the renal tumour, but the MRI scan (**726**) excludes it.

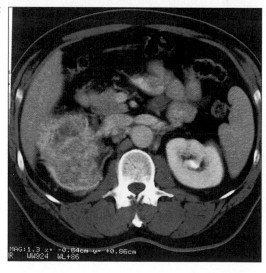

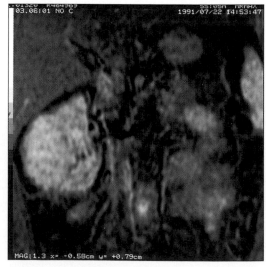

Chest radiography

727 Classical appearance of 'cannon ball' metastases seen throughout both lung fields.

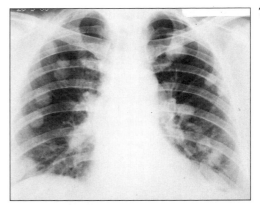

727

Bone metastases

728 Metastasis in the bone.

729 Pathological fracture in a weight-bearing bone.

728 729

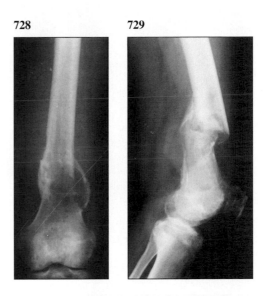

730 731

Sclerotic bone metastases in renal cortical carcinomas can be shown by bone scan.

730 demonstrates a large osteogenic metastasis in the body of the twelfth thoracic vertebra. A faint right renal outline can be seen to be distorted by the primary tumour.

MRI studies can also be helpful, particularly when secondaries involve the spinal column.

731 Metastasis from a renal cortical carcinoma involving the dorsal spine showing the collapsed vertebra and a soft tissue mass compressing the cord. There is also an enormous soft tissue deposit in the anterior mediastinum.

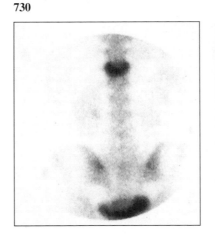

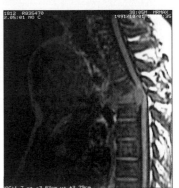

'Spontaneous regression'

A well-recognised, but rare, phenomenon occurs with the metastases from renal cortical tumours. After removal of the primary, pulmonary metastases can regress completely and bony metastases can recalcify without further treatment.

732

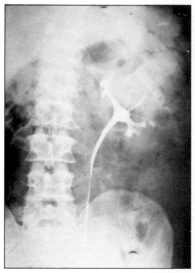

733

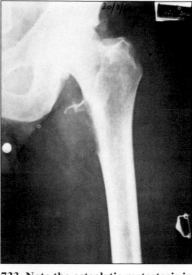

734

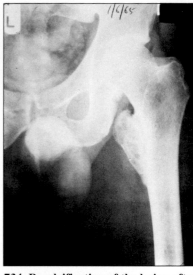

732 IVU of a renal carcinoma.

733 Note the osteolytic metastasis in the left lesser trochanter of this patient.

734 Recalcification of the lesion after nephrectomy, with no local treatment of the metastasis. The patient remains well and disease-free 17 years after surgery.

Typical renal tumours

735

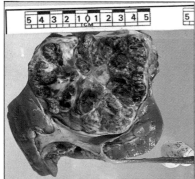

735 Renal cortical carcinoma. A large tumour distorting the pelvis and destroying much of the middle of the kidney. It is apparently encapsulated, and fibrous bands separate lobulated tumour masses.

736

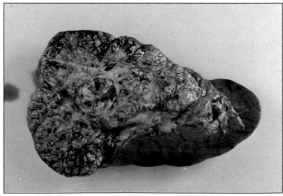

736 Renal cortical carcinoma. The whole of the lower pole is occupied by the tumour mass which has invaded the pelvis and extended through the capsule of the kidney.

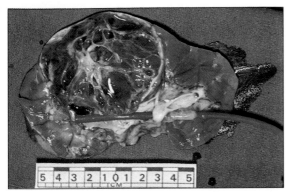

737 Renal cortical carcinoma. This apparently encapsulated cystic mass is actually a renal cortical carcinoma showing widespread cystic change.

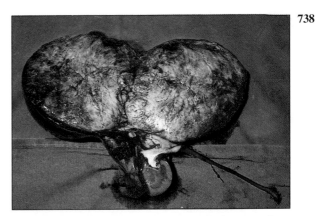

738 An encapsulated cortical tumour: a further example.

Renal cortical carcinoma

Renal cortical carcinoma is very variable in its appearance, even within the same tumour. Many patterns of cell growth can be recognised, but they are all variants of the same tumour, which arises from the tubular epithelial cell. The variable pattern makes this tumour particularly difficult to diagnose in a metastasis – a characteristic that has earned it the reputation of 'the great mimic'.

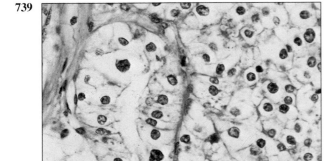

739 Clear-cell pattern. The tumour cells here look fairly regular and the cytoplasm of most of the cells is clear. There is some tubule formation. The clearness may be caused by intracellular lipid or glycogen. *(H&E × 256)*

740 Granular cells. A small vessel in the centre is surrounded by tumour cells, which have a rather granular cytoplasm. The granularity is a reflection of the many intracytoplasmic organelles in the cells of this pattern. *(H&E × 256)*

741 Papillary pattern. A tumour growing in a papillary pattern (i.e. the tumour cells are arranged as finger-like processes, which have a core of connective tissue and vessels covered with the malignant cells). *(H&E × 160)*

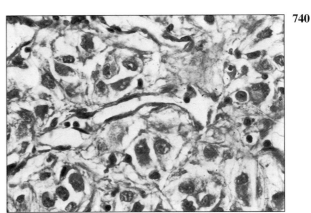

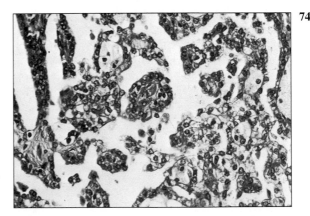

742

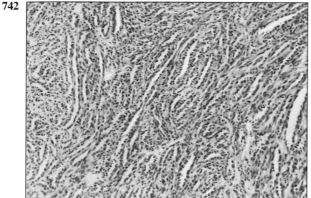

742 Tubular pattern. Tumour cells are arranged in a well-marked tubular pattern. *(H&E × 64)*

743

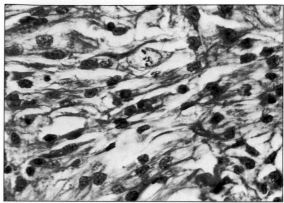

743 Spindle-cell pattern. Elongated tumour cells lie with their long axes parallel to each other. The appearances simulate those of a sarcoma rather than a carcinoma and may cause diagnostic difficulty, especially when the tumour presents as a metastatic deposit. Nevertheless, these cells can be shown to have epithelial characteristics. *(H&E × 256)*

744

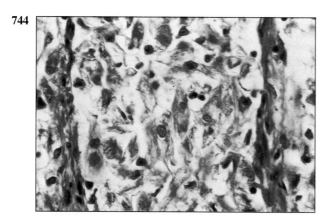

744 Vascular invasion. Tumour cells are seen in the lumen and surrounding a vein. This vascular invasion is a characteristic of renal cortical carcinoma and is associated with the high incidence of blood-borne metastases. *(H&E × 256)*

745

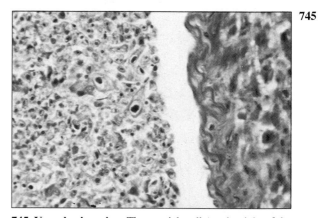

745 Vascular invasion. The arterial wall (on the right of the picture) abuts onto the tumour which has invaded into the lumen. The space between the wall and the tumour is an artefact caused by shrinking during processing. Vascular invasion and occlusion of the blood supply to a part of the tumour may be responsible for the high frequency of necrotic areas within the tumour. *(H&E × 160)*

746

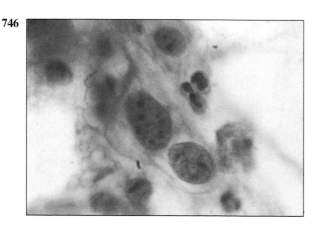

Aspiration biopsy

746 Cystic renal cortical carcinoma: cytology of needle aspirate. A clump of large cells in the middle of the field. The nuclei vary in size and the chromatin is irregularly clumped. The cytoplasm is plentiful, pale, and slightly foamy. A renal cortical carcinoma was subsequently removed. The cells with small lobed nuclei are polymorphonuclear leucocytes. *(H&E × 640)*

Oncocytoma

The presentation of the recently described entity of onco-cytoma is very similar to that of renal cortical carcinoma. However the appearances of oncocytomas and cortical tumours differ, particularly on CT and MRI studies, and the behaviour of oncocytoma is more benign.

747

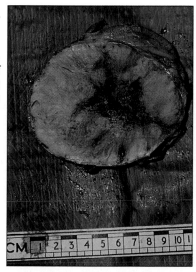

747 Macroscopic appearance of an oncocytoma.

748 Oncocytoma. High-power view of a section of an oncocytoma showing bland nuclei in eosinophilic cytoplasm. *(H&E × 256)*

748

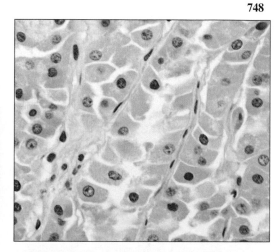

749

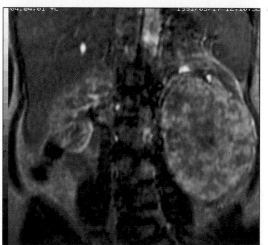

749 CT study after contrast shows the characteristic 'cartwheel' appearance of the oncocytoma.

750, 751 MRI studies before and after contrast show similar appearances.

750

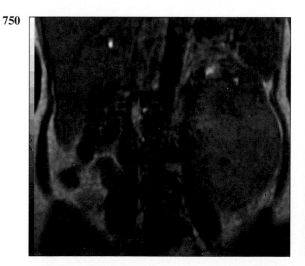

751

Adenomas

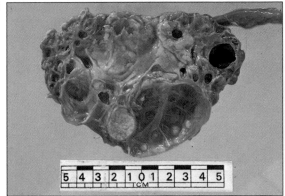

752 **A scarred cystic kidney** (acquired cystic disease following transplantation) in which there is a yellow nodule approximately 1.5 cm in diameter in the cortex. Adenomas have an appearance similar to that of well-differentiated adenocarcinomas. They are unlikely to cause metastases if they are less than 2 cm in diameter, provided the histology is benign. They tend to be chance findings.

753 **A microscopic adenoma**. The normal tubules are seen around the periphery of the field. In the centre is a small adenoma, showing a papillary structure and composed of hyperchromatic cells. *(H&E × 64)*

754 **Papillary pattern.** This picture contrasts normal tubular epithelium (lower right corner) and hyperchromatic cells arranged in a slightly papillary pattern in the adenoma. *(H&E × 160)*

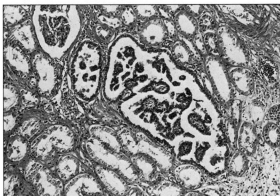

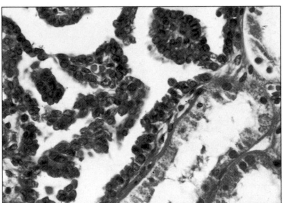

Nephroblastoma (Wilms' tumour)

Wilms' tumour is found exclusively in young children and commonly presents with abdominal swelling and finding of the mass. One-third of the children present with haematuria.

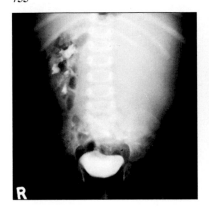

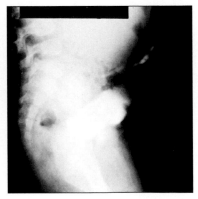

Intravenous urography

755 **Wilms' tumour.** A mass can be seen to occupy the whole of the left loin.

756 **Wilms' tumour**. A lateral film shows dye in the pelvis stretched over the tumour mass.

757 Wilms' tumour. A smaller tumour causing calyceal distortion and displacement on the IVU.

758 Wilms' tumour. Multiple metastases may occur and are very similar to those seen in patients with adult renal carcinoma.

757

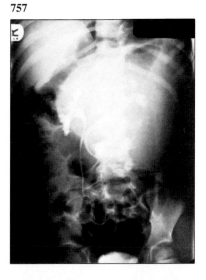

758

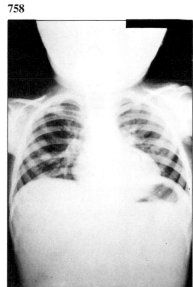

Wilms' tumours can extend through major vessels in the same way as patients with adult renal carcinoma.

759 MRI axial view of Wilms' tumour with involvement of the inferior vena cava by tumour extension into it.

760 MRI coronal view shows the extent of caval involvement.

759

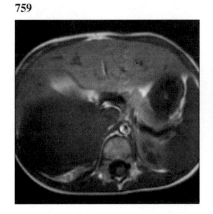

760

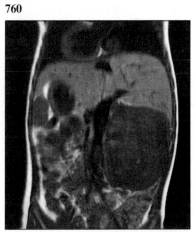

761 Section of Wilms' tumour in renal vein. Islands of cells with little cytoplasm are seen in the lumen of the vessel. *(H&E × 160)*

761

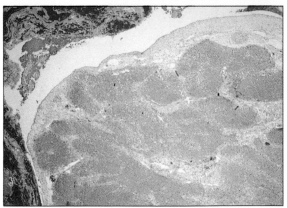

762

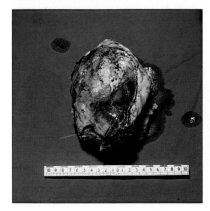

763

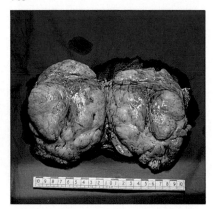

Examples of Wilms' tumour

762, 763 Wilms' tumour. The whole of the kidney has been destroyed by this pale fleshy mass.

Microscopic appearances of Wilms' tumour

764

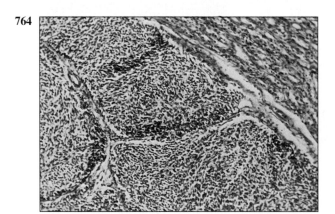

764 Tumour composed of sheets of small cells with dense nuclei and little cytoplasm. The normal renal parenchyma is seen at the top right hand corner of the picture. *(H&E × 64)*

765

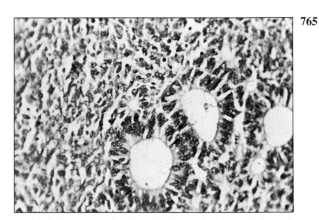

765 Higher magnification showing primitive tubules differentiating in a background of undifferentiated tumour. *(H&E × 160)*

766

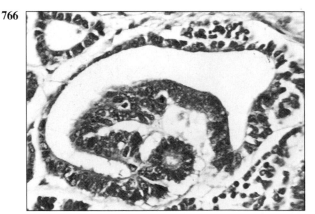

766 In some areas of the tumour, structures that resemble primitive glomeruli can occasionally be identified. *(H&E × 160)*

767

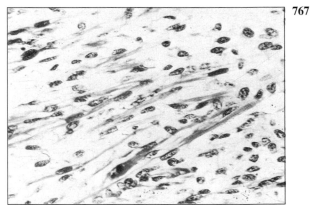

767 Area of tumour composed of elongated strap-like cells in which cross striations could be demonstrated. This is striated muscle differentiation in a nephroblastoma. *(H&E × 256)*

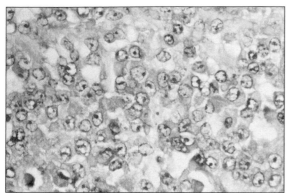

768 Rhabdoid tumour of the kidney is a malignant tumour seen particularly in infants and young children. It is distinct from nephroblastoma, but of uncertain histogenesis. Histologically it consists of large undifferentiated cells with vesicular nuclei containing one or two nucleoli and large eosinophilic cytoplasmic inclusions. The tumour does not form primitive glomeruli or tubules and nephrogenic rests are not seen. *(H&E × 256)*

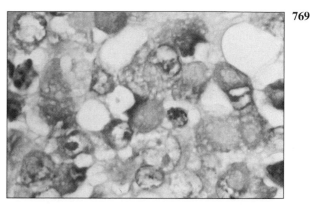

769 Rhabdoid tumour. A higher magnification demonstrates the characteristic eosinophilic inclusions. At electron microscopy these show large whorls of intermediate filaments. The tumour tends to be monomorphic, but there are several histological variants. *(H&E × 320)*

770 Congenital mesoblastic nephroma is the commonest renal tumour in infants up to 3 months of age. It is benign, but may recur if incompletely excised and occasional metastatic behaviour may occur when it presents in an older child. It is not usually encapsulated and the cut surface may have a whorled appearance similar to that of a leiomyoma. Histologically it is composed of plump spindle cells that have the characteristics of myofibroblasts or fibroblasts. Mitoses may be present, but high mitotic counts do not indicate malignancy in infants younger than 3 months. *(H&E × 256)*

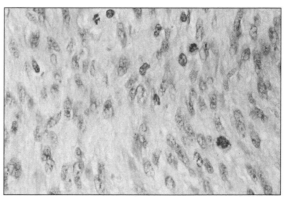

Leiomyosarcoma

771 Leiomyosarcoma. IVU showing abnormal calyceal pattern caused by a space-occupying lesion at the left lower pole.

772 Leiomyosarcoma. Arteriogram of the left kidney shows the classical appearance of microaneurysms similar to those seen in a hamartoma.

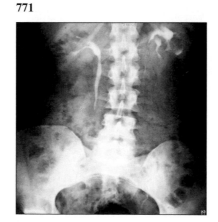

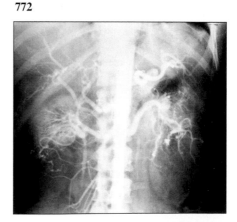

173

773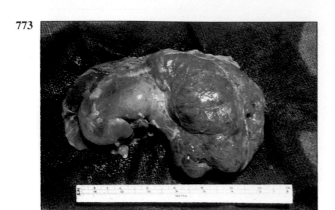

774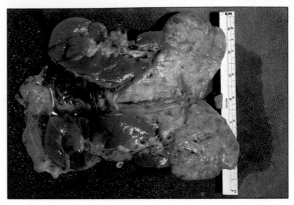

775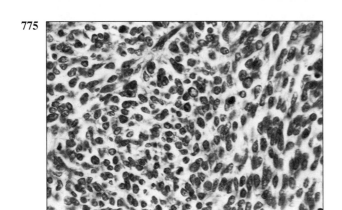

773, 774 An example of the rare leiomyosarcoma. A brown fleshy tumour mass occupying one pole of the kidney and invading through its capsule. This is usually a fatal condition but this patient remains alive and well 25 years later.

775 Leiomyosarcoma. Tumour composed of sheets of spindle cells with prominent mitotic figures. Ultrastructurally the cells have smooth muscle characteristics. *(H&E × 256)*

Angiomyolipoma

776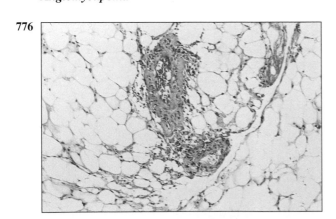

776 Angiomyolipoma is a hamartoma that contains tissue foreign to the part, and is therefore properly designated a choristoma. It is primarily a nonneoplastic overgrowth of adipose tissue, thick-walled blood vessels, and smooth muscle in varying proportions. Their developmental origin is shown by the fact that many patients with tuberous sclerosis have such lesions in the kidney, but they do occur in patients with no other manifestations of tuberous sclerosis. *(H&E × 64)*

777

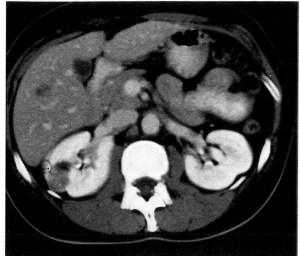

778

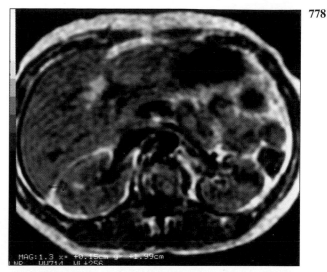

777 CT scan showing a filling defect in relation to a tumour arising in the right kidney.

778 MRI confirms that this is fat because of its high signal and therefore makes the diagnosis of angiomyolipoma.

Secondary carcinoma of the kidney

779 Secondary carcinoma of the kidney. This is a postmortem specimen showing a large metastasis in the kidney of a man who died as a result of carcinoma of the bronchus.

779

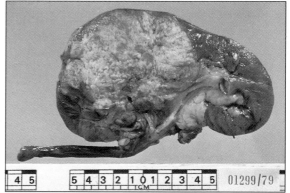

Lymphoma of the kidney

780 Lymphoma of the kidney. This is a postmortem specimen showing multiple small deposits of tumour in a man who died from a disseminated non-Hodgkin's lymphoma (diffuse, stem-cell type).

780

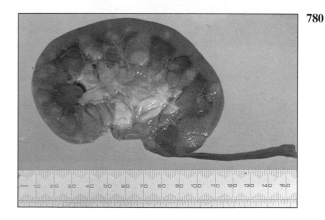

175

Cysts of the kidney (see also Chapter 2)

781

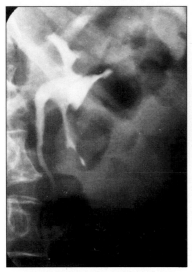

782

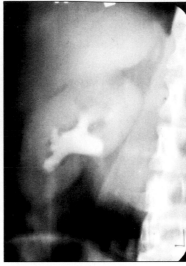

783

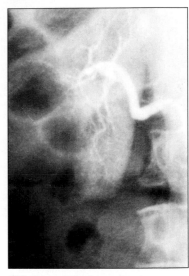

781 Cysts: IVU. The stretched calyceal distortion is indistinguishable from a solid space-occupying lesion.

782 Cysts: IVU. A space-occupying lesion in the upper pole.

783 Cysts: arteriography. An avascular area of the kidney with a well-demarcated edge.

784

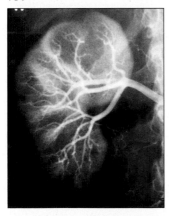

785

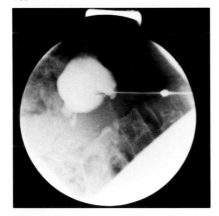

784 Cysts: arteriography. An avascular upper pole space-occupying lesion.

785 Cysts: puncture. Smooth internal surface of a cyst.

786

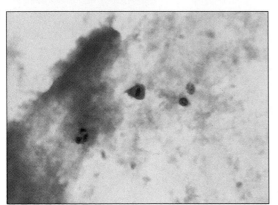

786 Cytology of this aspirate shows eosinophilic material in the background and a few isolated cells lacking any feature of malignancy. Compare with **746**. The cell with a lobed nucleus is a polymorphonuclear leucocyte. (*H&E × 256*)

Ultrasound and CT: comparative studies of cysts and renal cortical tumours

787 Ultrasound of longitudinal section of kidney shows a lower pole smooth-walled cyst with complete absence of any echoes.

788 For comparison, a longitudinal section of the contralateral kidney of the same patient reveals a complex mass of a similar size at the lower pole, which proved to be a tumour.

787

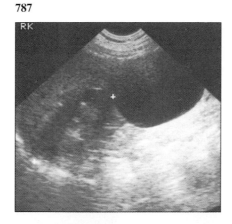

788

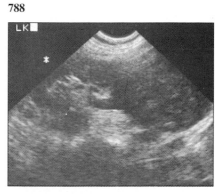

789

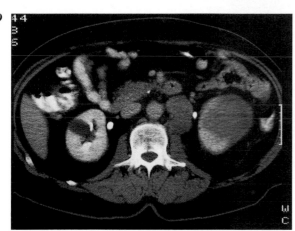

790

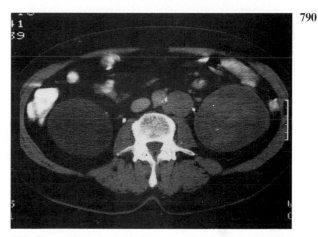

789 CT scanning of the same patient as in 787 and 788 shows a simple cyst of the right kidney and a mixed attenuation mass typical of a renal tumour on the left side.

790 Shows the presence of para-aortic glands on the left side.

791

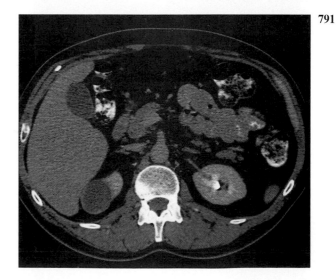

791 MRI confirms that the thick wall of the cyst in the right kidney is fibrous and not tumour.

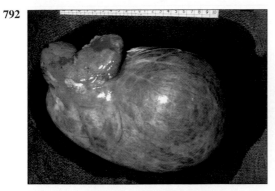

792 Macroscopic view of typical cyst showing the classic blue-domed appearance.

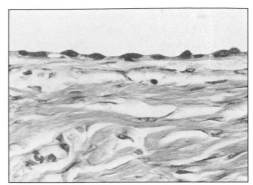

793 Cyst lined by a layer of flattened epithelium surrounded by fibrous tissue. *(H&E × 160)*

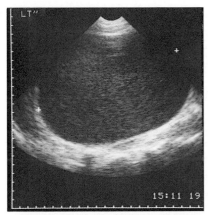

Cysts with intracystic malignancy can also develop.

794 Ultrasound study of a cystic kidney with bleeding into the cyst due to an underlying tumour.

795, 796 CTs demonstrating cystic tumour with solid tumour within the cyst.

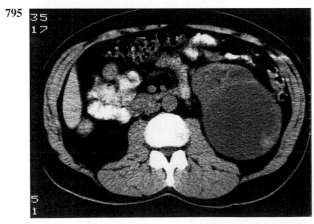

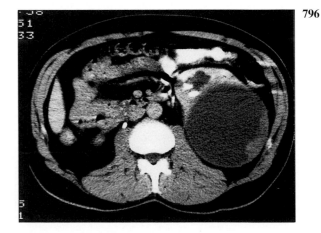

Renal cystic disease encompasses many types of renal abnormality. Multiple cysts are found in one or both kidneys without progressive destruction of the kidneys towards end renal failure.

797

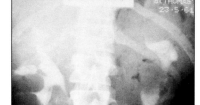

797 IVU showing bilateral enlarged kidneys with elongation of the calyces.

Arteriography

798, 799 Arteriograms of patient with multicysts. Multicystic disease of the kidney is frequently symptomless, but haematuria and renal pain may occur. In contradistinction, polycystic disease of the adult kidney is a genetically determined condition, which is bilateral and slowly progressive, often leading to hypertension and end-renal failure in adult life. Profuse haematuria may also occur, with loin pain when there is haemorrhage into the cysts.

798

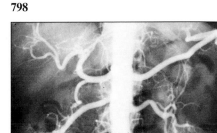

799

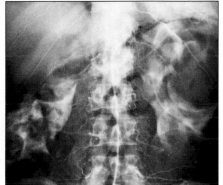

800

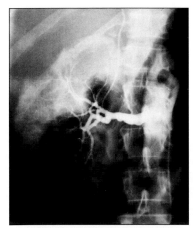

801

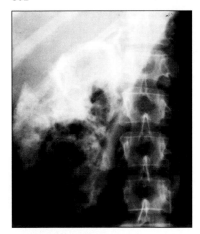

802

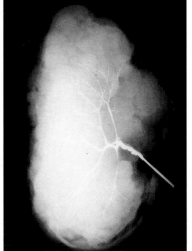

800, 801 Arteriogram confirms the presence of multiple cysts.

802 Arteriogram of excised specimen.

803

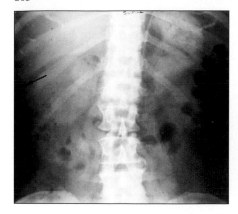

804

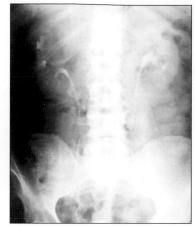

Investigation of a solitary benign cyst of kidney

803 Soft tissue swelling of right kidney (arrowed).

804 IVU of a space-occupying lesion.

805

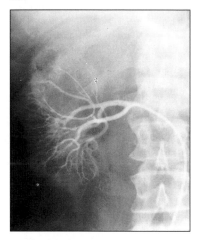

806

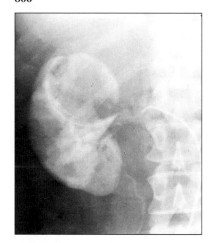

805 Selective renal arteriogram. Arterial phase outlines avascular cyst.

806 Venous phase of arteriogram: normal renal tissue surrounding cyst.

807

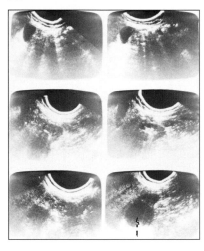

808

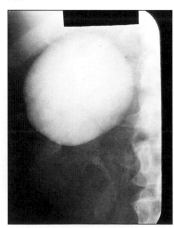

807 Ultrasound views confirm presence of cystic lesion (arrowed).

808 Cyst puncture: smooth internal surface of a benign cyst. See **794** for comparison showing a cyst with tumour within it.

Tumours of renal pelvis and ureter—TNM clinical classification

T (primary tumour)

TX Primary tumour cannot be assessed.
T0 No evidence of primary tumour.
Ta Papillary noninvasive carcinoma.
Tis Carcinoma *in situ*.
T1 Tumour invades subepithelial connective tissue.

T2 Tumour invades muscularis.
T3 Tumour invades beyond muscularis into peripelvic fat or renal parenchyma (renal pelvis). Tumour invades beyond muscularis into periureteric fat (ureter).
T4 Tumour invades adjacent organs or through the kidney into the perinephric fat.

N (regional lymph nodes)

N1 Single < 2 cm.
N2 Single > 2–5 cm, multiple < 5 cm.
N3 > 5 cm.

M (distant metastases)

M0 No metastases.
M1 Distant metastases.

Intravenous urography

Tumours arising in the calyces or renal pelvis produce filling defects easily visible on urography.

809

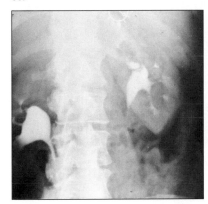

809 Tumour related to left upper calyx.

810

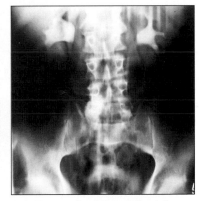

810 Tumour in right renal pelvis.

811

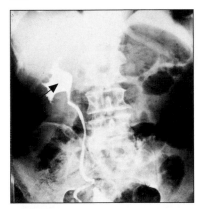

811 Filling phase. Lesion almost obscured (arrowed).

812

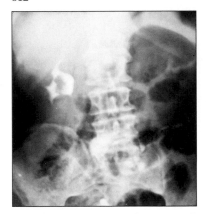

812 Emptying phase. Tumour well defined (macroscopic specimen **816**).

813

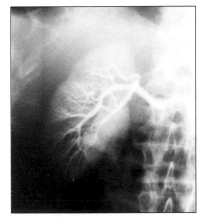

813 Arteriogram showing abnormal vascular pattern.

Ascending ureterography (**811, 812**) is invaluable for defining pelvic filling defects.

Arteriography (**813**) is usually normal, but occasionally pathological vessels can be seen in the region of the renal pelvis.

814

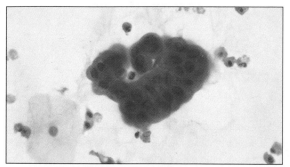

Urine cytology is often positive because these tumours are, in the main, transitional cell carcinomas.

814 Cytological examination of the urine is useful for detecting carcinoma of the renal pelvis and ureter. This specimen showed many clumps of cells like those in the centre of the field. They are transitional cells with some atypical features. The patient was shown to have a transitional cell carcinoma (see also **871** and **872**). (H&E × 256)

815

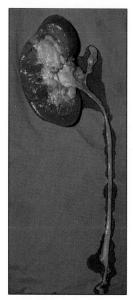

816

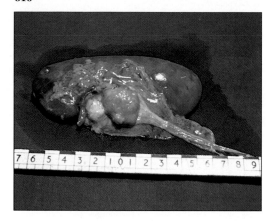

817

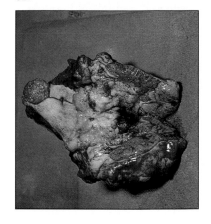

Transitional cell carcinoma of pelvis

815 Tumour arising in the pelvis in relation to the upper calyx is a papillary differentiated transitional cell carcinoma. No invasion was seen, but the renal parenchyma adjacent to the tumour showed fibrosis and chronic inflammatory changes.

816 Pelvis opened to show a rounded tumour sitting in the pelvis and growing into its lumen. This is a papillary differentiated transitional cell carcinoma.

817 Kidney opened to show a papillary tumour close to the pelviureteric junction. Proximal to this, the pelvis is dilated and the kidney shows scarring. These effects are caused by tumour obstruction.

818

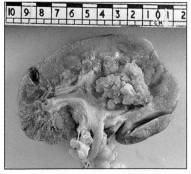

818 Papillary tumour. This specimen, which has been fixed in formalin and bisected, shows a papillary tumour involving the pelvis and calyceal system.

Ureteric tumours

Intravenous urography

Single or multiple tumours may appear as filling defects. Hydronephrosis and hydroureter may occur down to the level of the ureteric tumour.

819 Where complete ureteric stenosis occurs, nonfunction of that kidney will result.

Ascending ureterography

820 Ureteric tumours are well defined by retrograde studies.

Urine cytology

As with pelvic tumours, this is usually positive (see **814**).

821, 822 Hydronephrotic kidney caused by combined pelvic and ureteric tumours.

819

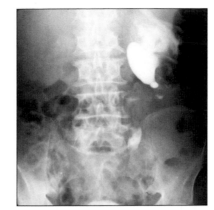

820

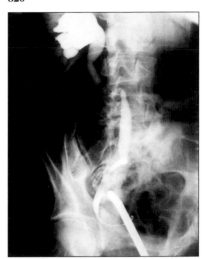

821

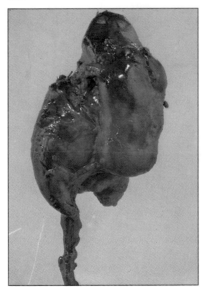

822

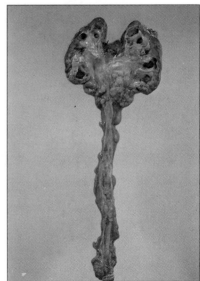

823

824

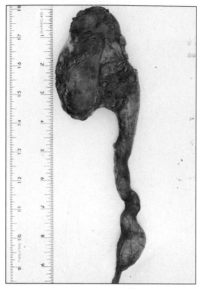

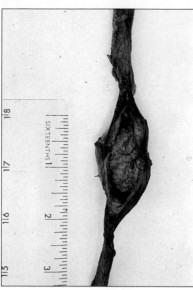

823, 824 Ureteric tumour obstructing ureter and resulting in hydroureter and hydronephrosis.

825

825 Positron emission tomography (PET). In the case shown here the patient had a tumour obstructing his lower ureter that was not amenable to biopsy. The question asked was 'Is there any tumour site other than that known that might be biopsied?' None was seen, and this was confirmed at surgery when an infiltrating tumour was found at the site indicated. It proved to be a poorly differentiated transitional cell carcinoma of the ureter with no abnormal para-aortic lymph nodes.

Transitional cell carcinoma of renal pelvis

These tumours have a similar histological appearance to carcinomas arising further down the urothelial tract.

Transitional cell carcinoma of ureter

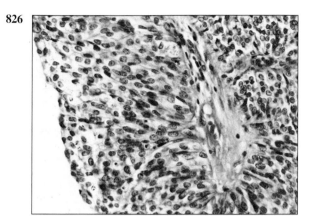

826 A section of a papillary differentiated transitional-cell carcinoma. *(H&E × 160)*

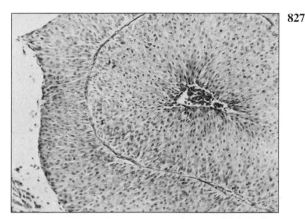

827 Histology of 823 and 824. A papillary differentiated transitional cell carcinoma.

Squamous carcinoma of renal pelvis

828 The kidney has a bifid pelvis. The calyces of the upper pole are filled by a calculus. Another calculus is lodged at the pelvic bifurcation and the calyces arising from the lower portion are dilated; the corresponding renal tissue is atrophied. A warty tumour is seen arising from the lining of these calyces. Histology showed a keratinising squamous carcinoma arising in squamous epithelium, associated with hydronephrosis and stones.

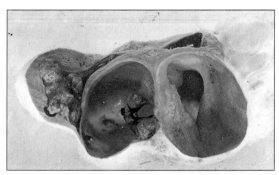

Squamous metaplasia of kidney

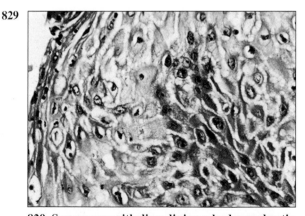

829 Squamous epithelium lining a hydronephrotic pelvis. This is squamous metaplasia (i.e. the type of epithelium has changed from a transitional to a squamous type). There are also some atypical changes in the cells. These changes often arise in association with calculi and infection. *(H&E × 256)*

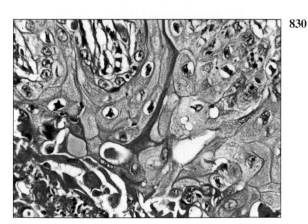

830 Sometimes carcinomas arising in the renal pelvis show squamous differentiation. This tumour shows large cells resembling those of the prickle cell layer of the skin and keratin formation. *(H&E × 256)*

831

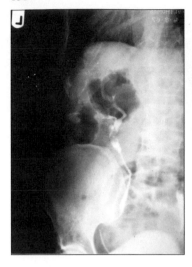

832

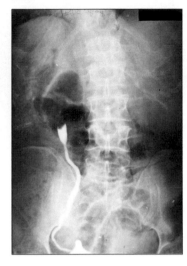

Ureteric polyp

831 IVU showing filling defect in ureter simulating carcinoma.

832 Ascending ureterography demonstrates the smooth meniscus effect. Again it is difficult to differentiate this from ureteric carcinoma.

833

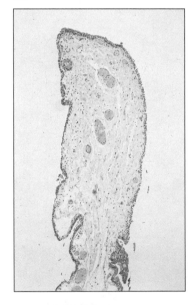

834

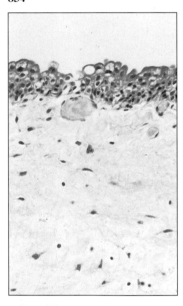

833 The polyp consists of a core of connective tissue and vessels covered with transitional epithelium. *(H&E × 26)*

834 A higher magnification of 833 showing the bland appearance of the epithelium and of the fibrous core. There is no evidence of malignancy and the lesion is best called a fibroepithelial polyp. *(H&E × 160)*

835

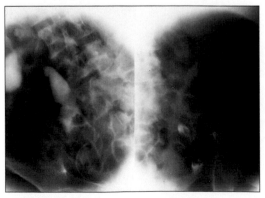

835 Bilateral ureteric tumour.

836

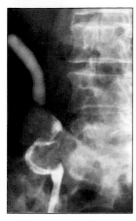

837

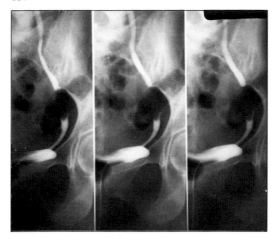

836, 837 Tumour filling defect. Retrograde studies also clearly delineate the ureteric filling defect of the tumour.

838

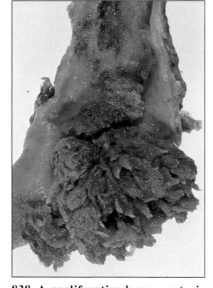

838 A proliferative lower ureteric carcinoma.

839

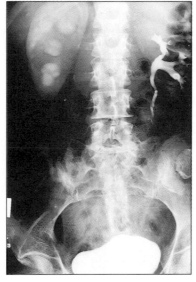

840

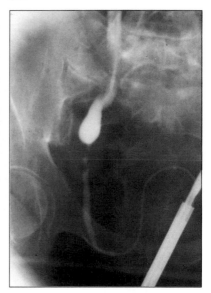

839, 840 Endometriosis may, rarely, obstruct the ureter producing ureteric obstruction by stricture. The IVU (**839**) demonstrates the markedly obstructed kidney and an ascending study (**840**) shows the stricture low down in the ureter within the bony pelvis.

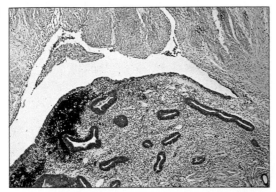

841 Ureteric endometriosis. In the lower part of the field there is a tumour-like mass composed of glands and stroma. This is endometriosis. These glands can be misdiagnosed as adenocarcinoma by the unwary. They may show mitoses, but lack other features of malignancy. The stroma is the clue.

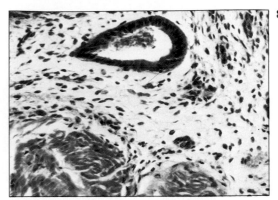

842 Endometriosis. A higher magnification shows an endometrial gland with its loose stroma, the combination constituting endometriosis. The diagnosis cannot be made without identifying glands and stroma. Ureteric smooth muscle is seen at the bottom of the field.

Renal artery stenosis

Hypertension may accompany many forms of renal disease, particularly when it is unilateral. Although uncommon, renal artery disease is well recognised as a cause of renal hypertension. Atheromatous plaques within the lumen, and fibromuscular disorders of the vessel itself are the mechanisms of this process. Renal size is frequently reduced on the side of the lesion.

The classical pyelographic findings are those of delay in excretion on the affected side with relatively increased concentration in later films caused by slow transit through the kidney. Divided renal function studies have now been largely replaced by renography and renal scans. Measurements of plasma renin or angiotensin are often used. A ratio of plasma renin activity from the stenosed versus the contralateral kidney exceeding 1.5 is felt to be significant in most cases in assessment of the effects of the stenosis.

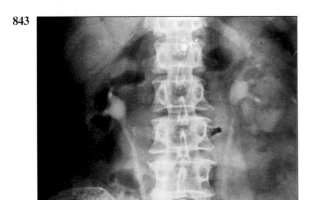

843 IVU of a patient with hypertension reveals a smaller right kidney with increased concentration of the dye on that side.

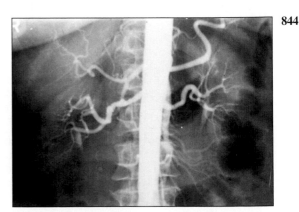

844 Flood renal arteriogram: classical fibromuscular hyperplasia of the right renal artery.

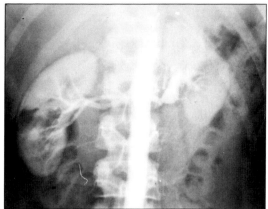

845 Post-stenotic dilatation of this left renal artery caused by an atheromatous stricture.

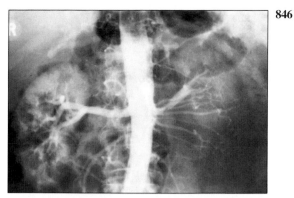

846 Another left-sided stricture with an associated small kidney.

847 Bilateral arterial disease is present and is more pronounced on the left.

848 A normal standard dynamic renal scan and renogram using I^{123} hippuran.
  Divided function
  L/L+R = 62%

849 The normal renogram pattern is worsened by captopril therapy and shows a positive scan for renal artery stenosis. Captopril, an angiotensin-converting enzyme inhibitor, relaxes the efferent glomerular arterioles and reduces filtration pressure, which increases functional impairment as measured by renography.
  Divided function
  L/L+R = 77%

—— = Left
········· = Right
——— = Blood

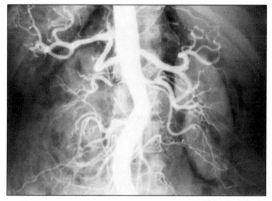

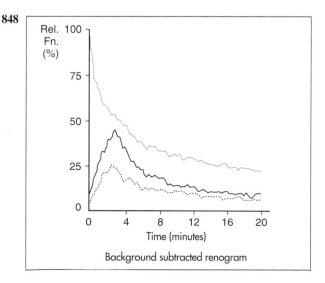

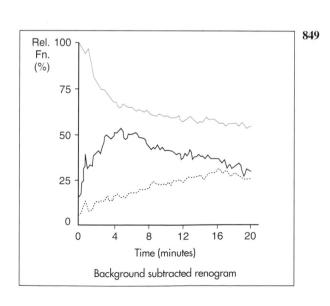

850

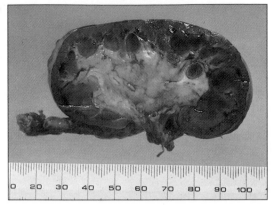

850 Renal artery stenosis. Nephrectomy specimen. This hemisection shows a small kidney with a narrowed cortex associated with a renal artery stenosis. This kidney does not show gross scarring.

851

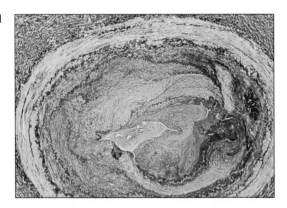

851 Renal artery stenosis. Section through a renal artery showing fibroelastic internal proliferation resulting in marked narrowing of the lumen. *(Elastic van Gieson)*

852

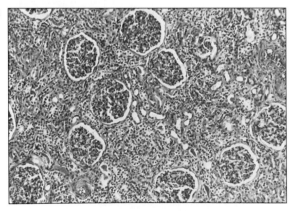

852 Renal artery stenosis. Section through the cortex showing glomeruli surviving among atrophic tubules. Glomeruli are crowded together because of the tubular atrophy. *(H&E × 64)*

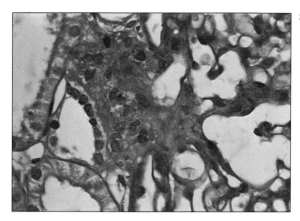

853 Renal artery stenosis. When glomerular ischaemia is present there is often hyperplasia of the juxtaglomerular apparatus (arrow). This group of cells is found at the hilum of the glomerulus. It is made up of cells of the afferent arterioles, the macula densa of the distal convoluted tubule, and the cells of Goormaghtigh, which are continuous with the cells of the glomerular mesangium on the right of the field. *(PAS × 400)*

Renal trauma

Renal trauma as a result of penetrating injuries and blunt trauma is becoming more common. If there may have been renal injury as a result of penetrating wounds, an IVU is the first-line investigation. Evidence of nonfunction on the side of the trauma is highly suggestive of injury to the vascular pedicle and demands immediate exploration. Blunt trauma, often in relation to road traffic accidents, can produce a varying degree of renal damage and can be assessed with CT and arteriography.

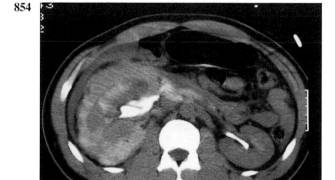
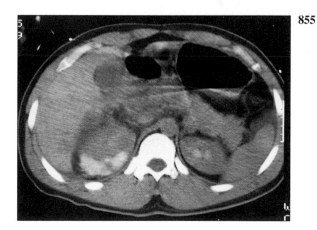

854, 855 CT studies showing a gross perirenal haematoma with contrast extravasation. Contrast in the collecting system indicates that the kidney still functions.

856

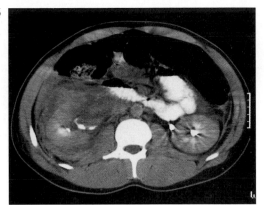

857

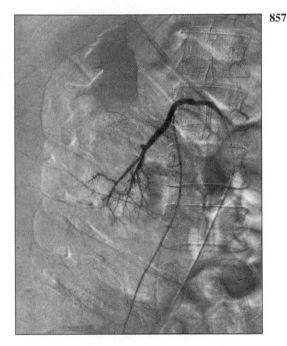

856 A further study 4 days later shows an improvement in the nephrogram and less extravasation of contrast.

857 A digital subtracted arteriogram taken a further 5 days later demonstrates the lower pole artery supplying the lower moiety of the kidney, which has been separated from the body of the organ by the trauma.

8 Bladder tumours

The investigation and treatment of bladder tumours take up a major portion of a urologist's time. Advances in therapy of this complex subject have been slow and unspectacular, but a better recognition of the many aspects of the problem has allowed urologists to be more specific and precise in their approach to the different types of tumour. If this approach is to be progressive, a pathological classification is essential.

858 Classification of urinary bladder tumours.

I Epithelial	Benign	Transitional cell papilloma Inverted type of transitional cell papilloma Squamous papilloma
	Malignant	Transitional cell papilloma Squamous cell carcinoma Adenocarcinoma Undifferentiated carcinoma
II Non-epithelial	Benign	Soft-tissue lesions, e.g. leiomyoma
	Malignant	Rhabdomyosarcoma Others, e.g. leiomyosarcoma
III Miscellaneous	e.g.	Phaecochromocytoma, lymphoma, carcinosarcoma, malignant melanoma

About 95% of bladder tumours are epithelial in origin and in Western countries about 95% of these are transitional cell type. Carcinomas are further characterised in terms of growth pattern (papillary or solid, or both), histological grading (degree of differentiation), staging (extent of spread), and type of spread.

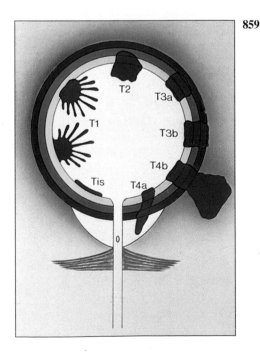

859 Diagrammatic representation of the classification adapted from the UICC. The UICC classification enables the clinician to describe and record bladder tumour data in internationally accepted terms. The extent or 'stage' of the primary tumour (T) with assessment of the presence or absence of local spread (T 1–4), lymphatic (N) and distant metastases (M) can thus be described. The pathologist will then examine any available tissue to determine the extent of spread of the disease or histopathological stage (P), and microscopy will demonstrate the histopathological grade or degree of differentiation of the primary tumour (G).

Classification of tumours

The meaning of TNM symbols are as follows:
- **T**: Clinical examination, urography, cystoscopy, bimanual examination under full anaesthesia, and biopsy or transurethral resection of the tumour before definitive treatment.
- **N**: Clinical examination, lymphography, and urography.
- **M**: Clinical examination, chest X-ray, and biochemical tests and the more advanced primary tumours or when clinical suspicion warrant, radiographic isotope studies.

Classification as applied to bladder tumours

T (primary tumour)

Tls Pre-invasive carcinoma, carcinoma *in situ*, 'flat tumour'.

Ta Papillary noninvasive carcinoma.

Tx The minimum requirements to assess the extent of the primary tumour fully cannot be met.

T0 No evidence of primary tumour.

T1 On bimanual examination a freely mobile mass may be felt. This should not be felt after complete transurethral resection of the lesion and/or microscopically the tumour does not extend beyond the lamina propria.

T2 On bimanual examination there is induration of the bladder wall, which is mobile. There is no residual induration after complete transurethral resection of the lesion and/or there is microscopic invasion of superficial muscle.

T3 On bimanual examination induration or a nodular mobile mass is palpable in the bladder wall, which persists after transurethral resection of the exophytic part of the lesion and/or there is microscopic invasion of deep muscle or of extension through the bladder wall.

    T3a Invasion of deep muscle.

    T3b Invasion through the bladder wall.

T4 Tumour fixed or invading neighbouring structures and/or there is microscopic evidence of such an involvement.

    T4a Tumour invading prostate, uterus, or vagina.

    T4b Tumour fixed to the pelvic wall and/or infiltrating the abdominal wall.

N (regional and juxtaregional lymph nodes)

N0 No evidence of regional lymph node involvement.

N1 Evidence of involvement of a single homolateral regional lymph node.

N2 Evidence of involvement of contralateral or bilateral or multiple regional lymph nodes.

N3 Evidence of involvement of fixed regional lymph nodes (there is a fixed mass on the pelvic wall with a free space between this and the tumour).

N4 Evidence of involvement of juxtaregional lymph nodes.

NX The minimum requirements to assess the regional and/or juxtaregional lymph nodes cannot be met.

M (distant metastases)

M0 No evidence of distant metastases.

M1 Evidence of distant metastases.

MX The minimum requirements to assess the presence of distant metastases cannot be met.

pTNM (postsurgical histopathological classification)

Staging may be carried out by the pathologist. Histopathological categories show the extent of tumour spread.

● **P**: An assessment of the P categories is based on evidence derived from surgical operation and histopathology (i.e. when a tissue other than biopsy is available for examination).

● **G**: Histopathological grading, which is a measure of the degree of differentiation of the tumour.

Pls Pre-invasive carcinoma, carcinoma *in situ*.
Px The extent of invasion cannot be assessed.
P0 No tumour found on examination of specimen.
Pl Tumour not extending beyond the lamina propria.

P2 Tumour with infiltration of superficial muscle not more than halfway through the muscle coat.
P3 Tumour with invasion of deep muscle more than halfway through the muscle coat or infiltration of perivesical tissue.
P4 Tumour with infiltration of prostate or other extravesical strictures.

Gx Grade cannot be assessed.
G0 No evidence of anaplasia (i.e. papilloma).
G1 Low-grade malignancy (see UICC definitions).
G2 Medium-grade malignancy (see UICC definitions).
G3 High-grade malignancy (see UICC definitions).

Histological examples of the various grades of tumours

Grade 1

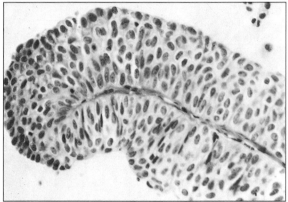

860 Papillary transitional cell carcinoma. This tumour has approximately seven layers of closely packed transitional cells covering a fibrovascular core. *(H&E × 160)*

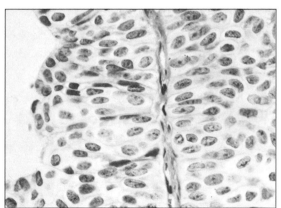

861 Papillary transitional cell carcinoma. Higher magnification of **860** showing the slight variation in size and shape of the transitional cells. *(H&E × 256)*

Grade 2

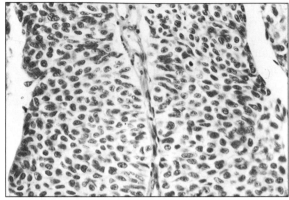

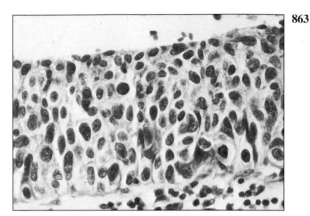

862 Papillary transitional cell carcinoma. This tumour has approximately 12 layers of closely packed transitional cells covering a fibrovascular core. *(H&E × 160)*

863 Papillary transitional cell carcinoma. Higher magnification of another area of **862** showing the moderate pleomorphism of the transitional cells. *(H&E × 256)*

Grade 3

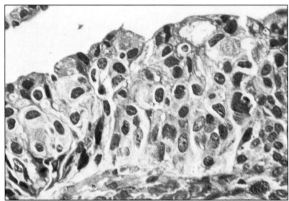

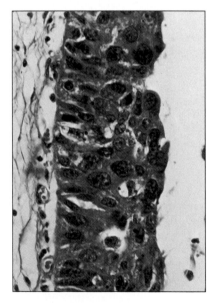

864 Transitional cell carcinoma. These cells show considerable pleomorphism. It is difficult to tell that they are transitional cells. *(H&E × 256)*

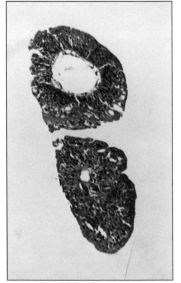

865 Carcinoma *in situ*. This is a section from a flat (i.e. nonpapillary) lesion in the bladder wall. The thickening of the epithelium and cellular atypia is such that it must be regarded as a carcinoma *in situ*. *(H&E × 160)*

Most papillary lesions in the bladder are papillary transitional cell carcinomas. Lesions classified as papillomas show no histological evidence of malignancy.

Simple papilloma is rare. It is small with a thin stalk, usually single, with very few fronds. Multiple bladder biopsies rarely reveal any additional tumours and the common presenting symptom is painless haematuria.

866 Histological appearance. The simple papilloma is covered with normal transitional epithelium. It shows no atypia, thickening or mitotic figures. *(H&E × 26)*

867 Bladder. Section through a simple papilloma. Its structure is that of a simple finger-like outgrowth. This is a core of connective tissue covered with normal transitional epithelium. *(H&E original mag. × 256)*

868 Inverted papilloma. These uncommon lesions are usually recognised at endoscopy. Histology reveals their architecture, which is that of a polyp with a smooth outer surface covering a mass of interconnecting trabeculae of transitional cells. *(H&E × 26)*

867

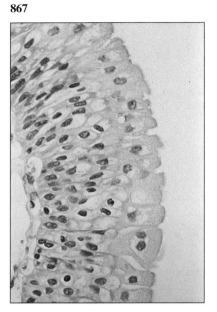

868

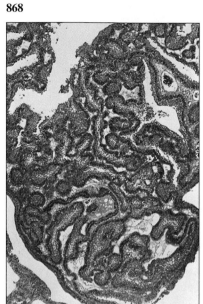

869 Inverted papilloma. Higher powered section showing the surface epithelium. These lesions appear to be benign, but one has to be very sure that one is not dealing with a transitional cell carcinoma. *(H&E × 64)*

870 Papillary transitional cell carcinoma. Section through the fronds of a papillary transitional cell carcinoma to show its architecture. *(H&E original mag. × 64)*

869

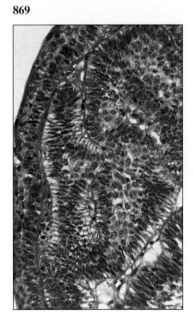

870

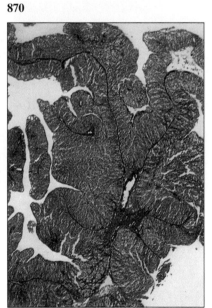

871

872

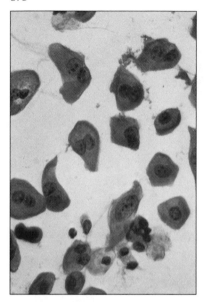

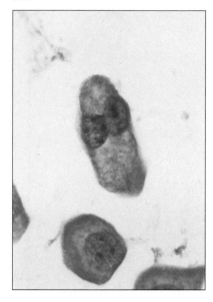

871 Urine cytology. Many atypical transitional cells, some multinucleate, from the urine of a patient with a transitional cell carcinoma of the bladder. *(H&E original mag. × 256)*

872 Urine cytology. Higher magnification showing the abnormal chromatin pattern in the nucleus of the transitional cells. *(H&E original mag. × 640)*

873

874

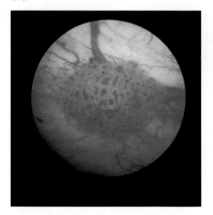

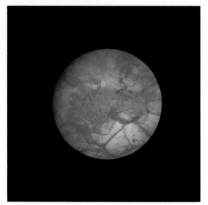

873 Discrete small papillary T1 tumour with normal surrounding bladder mucosa. The fronded appearance can be seen.

874 A less well-confined low-papillary T1 tumour showing the confluent appearance of this multifocal process.

875

876

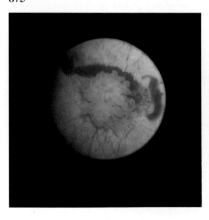

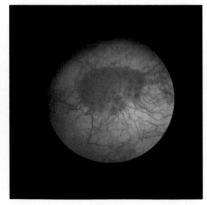

Haemorrhage close to a tumour is not infrequently seen and is due to trauma to a small vessel in one of the superficial fronds.

875 T1 tumour with a surrounding clot caused by haemorrhage.

876 Further example of T1 tumour.

877

877, 878 The same T1 tumour examined by rigid (**877**) and by flexible (**878**) cystoscopy.

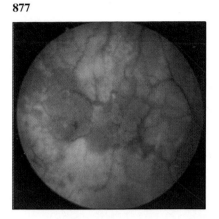

878

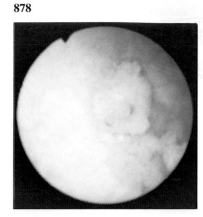

Histology of P1 tumour

879 P1 tumour showing invasion of lamina propria to be the deepest extent of the tumour. *(H&E × 256)*

879

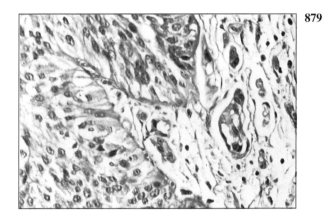

T2 tumours

These tumours may be small or large enough to fill the whole bladder. They may be round and tufted, showing short stunted fronds and have a broad base. Some have a wide pedicle, which is difficult to see because of the exuberance of the tufts near the base of the tumour. Others have long delicate fimbrial tissue up to 2.5 cm in length, which wave and swirl in the fluid medium like a bunch of seaweed. Sometimes the ends of the villae become avascular and their colour becomes either pale yellow or glistening white.

880

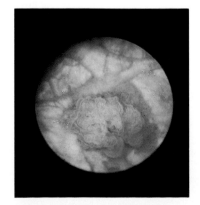

880 A rounded tufted tumour.

881

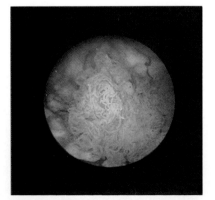

881 Sessile tumour on the base of the bladder.

882

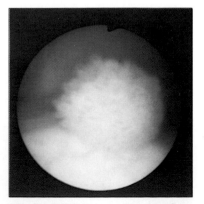

882 Sessile tumour as viewed by flexible cystoscopy.

883

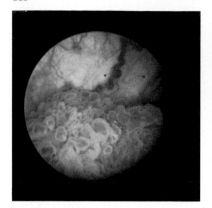

884

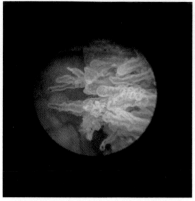

885

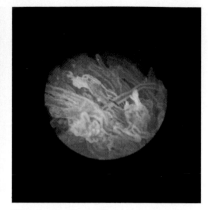

883 A similar tumour showing increased vascularity.

884 A typical long-fronded tumour. These tumours are large and it is always difficult to see the base, which may be very narrow.

885 Avascular tufts at the end of long fronds.

An IVU often provides valuable information.

886

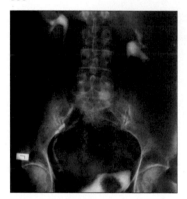

887

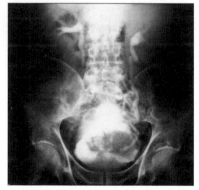

888

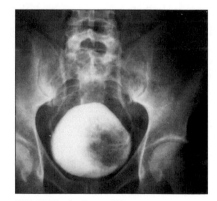

886 IVU showing round filling defect in the bladder.

887 IVU of large superficial tumour anterior to the ureteric orifice. This is not involved as the ureter is clearly shown behind tumour causing the filling defect.

888 IVU of a large T2 tumour showing the villous structure and the absence of penetration as the bladder outline is smooth and regular.

889

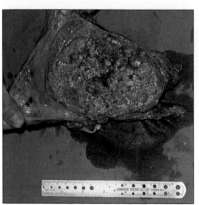

890

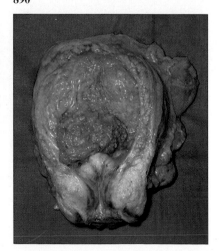

889 Specimen of T2 tumour filling the bladder.

890 Large T2 tumour with a coincidental prostatic enlargement, especially the middle lobe. It has a wide base and when the bladder was intact filled a large area of the cavity.

891 CT scanning is also extremely valuable in the assessment of the stage of tumours. Here a tumour can be seen arising from around the left ureteric orifice and obstructing the ureteric orifice itself.

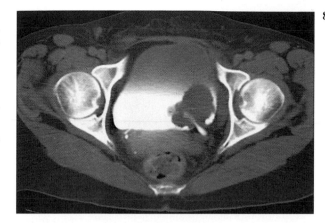

891

Bladder tumours may be one manifestation of numerous tumours involving any part of the urothelium. Multiple tumours of the renal tract occur in 10% of all cases of bladder tumour. It is mandatory to undertake a careful examination of the ureter and renal pelvis in all cases of bladder tumour, and a bilateral ureterogram using a bulb catheter should be performed. On rare occasions bladder tumours may present at one of the ureteric orifices and have a thin pedicle.

892

893

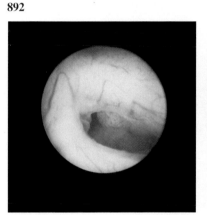

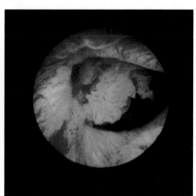

892 Tumour appearing in a dilated ureteric orifice. Such tumours are small and move in and out with each jet of urine. Another rare presentation is at the bladder neck.

893 Tumour involving the bladder neck. Note the pedunculated base and the long fronds. Tumours seen in this area are usually one of many other tumours spread over the surface of the bladder.

Histology of P2 tumours

894 P2 tumour. Transitional cell tumour invading the superficial muscle. *(H&E × 160)*

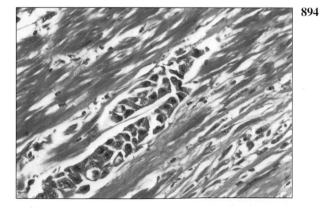

894

895

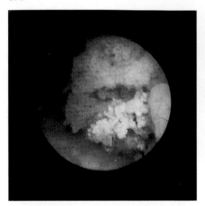

896

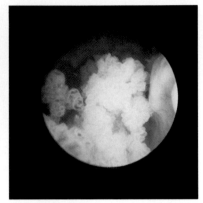

Endoscopic appearance of T3a tumour

These tumours are irregular and single and may have a surface slough. Presenting symptoms are haemorrhage, dysuria, frequency, and occasional straining due to superimposed secondary infection.

895 Infiltrating papillary tumour with some superficial haemorrhage and necrosis.

896 Infiltrating papillary tumour. A similar tumour with a larger area of surface slough.

Histology of P3 tumours

897

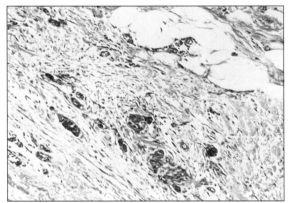

898

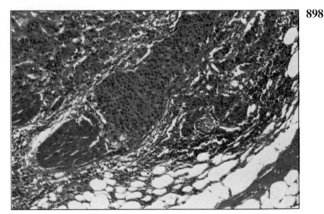

897 P3 tumour invading deep muscle. *(H&E × 32)*

898 P3b tumour showing invasion of perivesical fat. *(H&E × 64)*

899

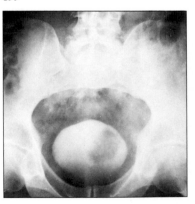

900

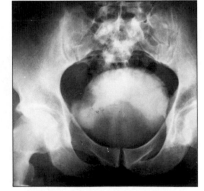

Just as with T2 tumours an IVU is a great help.

899 IVU of a T3a tumour invading muscle. The tumour involves the complete thickness of the muscle so that the outline is irregular.

900 IVU of a small T3a tumour with total muscle invasion. This picture also shows a bladder filling defect caused by an enlarged prostate.

901

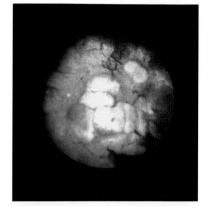

Endoscopic appearance of T3b tumour

It is impossible to differentiate between T3a and T3b on the endoscopic appearance.

901 Sessile nodular infiltrating tumour showing superficial necrosis, oedema, and inflammation of the surrounding tissues.

902 Extensive nodular infiltrating tumour with early ulceration.

903 Any T3b tumour can appear as a massive irregular growth with papilliferous formation. Here the villi are necrotic and ulcerated and appear as white, almost transparent, tissue.

904 A T3b tumour, which is nodular and adenomatous and has superficial slough. The brown areas are caused by submucosal blood pigments.

902

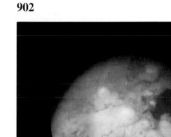

903

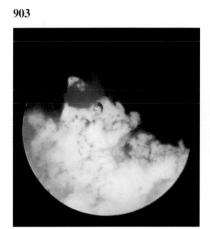

904

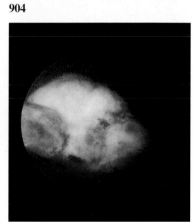

An IVU may give valuable information, especially when there is involvement of one or other ureteric orifices.

905

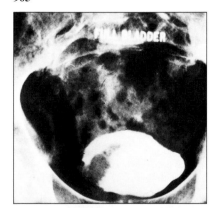

906

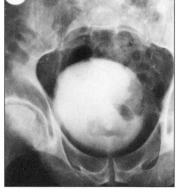

907

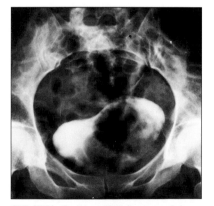

905 IVU of a small T3b tumour invading the bladder wall, where there is a complete gap in the bladder contour.

906 Further IVU of a larger T3b tumour invading the bladder wall.

907 IVU of a large T3b tumour. A large part of the bladder has been destroyed.

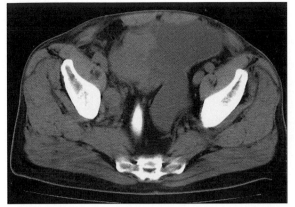

908 CT scan of T3 bladder tumour. This also shows an enlarged right iliac lymph node. Note the posterior diverticulum, which is not involved with tumour.

909 IVU of a large T3b tumour involving the left side of the bladder.

910 Multiple T3b tumours, one of which is involving the right ureter.

911 T3b tumour with early involvement of one ureter of a duplex system causing hydronephrosis. The upper ureter is involved causing dilatation of the lower renal moiety.

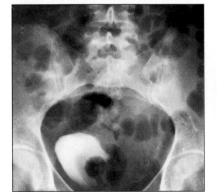

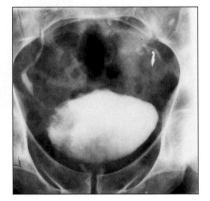

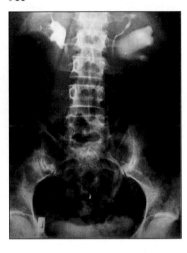

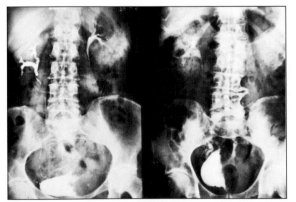

The intravenous urographic appearance may be a reliable method of assessing the invasive property of a bladder tumour.

912 A combination of two urograms, both showing extensive bladder involvement. One is a low-grade noninvasive tumour (T2) that has not affected the upper urinary tract, while the other is an aggressive invasive growth (T3a or T3b) that has caused a complete obstruction of the ureter.

913

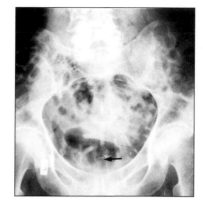

913 On rare occasions bladder tumours become calcified. An area of speckled calcification involves a tumour on the left side of the base of the bladder. This is usually a T3b or T4 tumour.

914

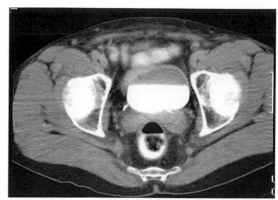

914 CT scan of T3 bladder tumour.

Endoscopic appearances of T4 tumours

The endoscopic appearances are indistinguishable from T3b tumours, but the lesions tend to be more extensive and ulceration is more common. The following four pictures show all the characteristics—ulceration, infiltration, inflammation, and oedema.

915

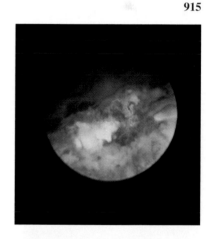

915 Irregular form with an amorphous appearance on section. No normal mucous membrane is seen and on bimanual examination the bladder wall feels thickened and indurated with extension into the paravesical tissues.

916

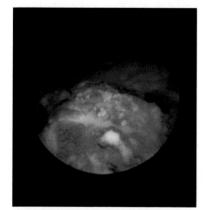

916 Ulcerated tumour surface. There is superimposed inflammation, manifest by granulation tissue spreading onto the bladder.

917

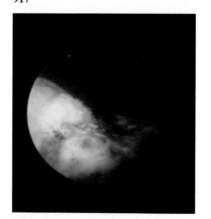

917 Tumour haemorrhage. Some tumours have altered blood pigments on the surface, which implies haemorrhage into the tumour.

918

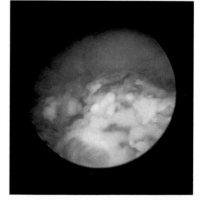

918 Tumour calcification. Another appearance is a white area caused by calcification, which is well shown in this picture.

919

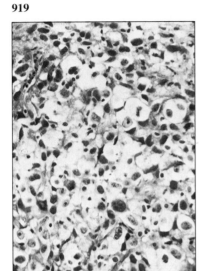

920

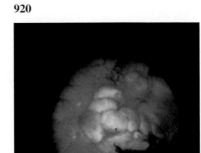

919 Undifferentiated carcinoma. This solid invasive tumour lacks differentiating features by which one can identify it as being of transitional cell origin. *(H&E × 256)*

920 Undifferentiated carcinoma. The endoscopic appearances are indistinguishable from a T3a or T3b tumour, but the nodular appearance shown here is often seen.

Advanced T4 tumours can invade surrounding bone.

921

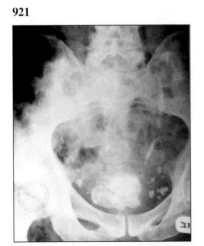

922

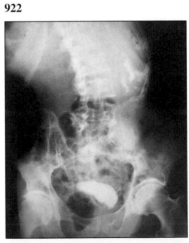

923

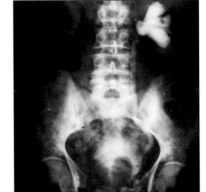

921, 922 Undifferentiated carcinoma. An anteroposterior and lateral IVU of T4 tumour. The tumour was palpable and fixed to the pelvic wall. It may be difficult to differentiate between T3b and T4 tumours by this investigation.

923 Undifferentiated carcinoma. IVU showing not only involvement of the left ureter, but also destruction of part of the pubic and ischial bones.

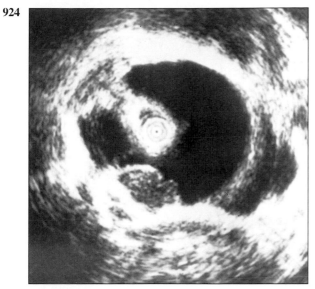

924 An ultrasound recording demonstrates an unsuspected tumour at the mouth of a diverticulum. With further experience staging of bladder tumours may be possible with ultrasound.

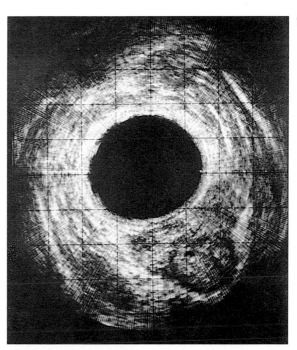

925 Normal bladder outline.

It has not been possible to achieve the complete diagnostic potential of ultrasound for bladder scanning. However, with recent developments it is now possible to introduce the transducer into the bladder through the cystoscope. The transducer head can be rotated through a 360° circle to perform a semirenal time scan and allows accurate diagnosis of different bladder tumours.

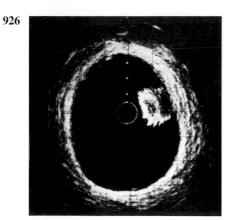

926 T1 tumour.

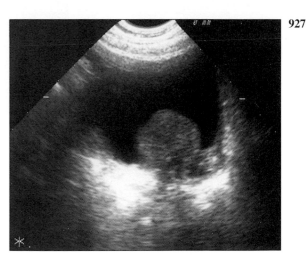

927 Ultrasound of large T2 bladder tumour. Note that there is no evidence of any projected shadow as seen with a similar size stone (see **656**, p.149).

928

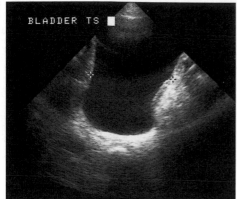

929

928 Scan of T2 bladder tumour.

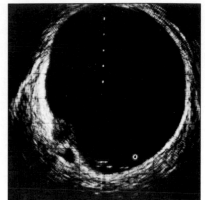

929 Scan of T3a or T3b tumour.

Metastases

As well as local spread the tumour can involve the liver. Very occasionally bones are involved.

930

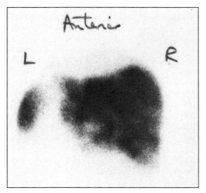

931

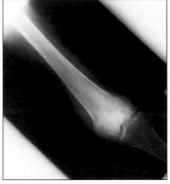

932

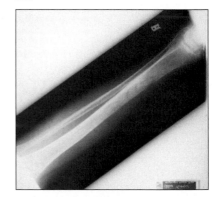

930 Scan of a liver containing multiple metastases, manifested by increased uptake of ^{99m} Tc.

931 Early metastases in femoral condyle.

932 Early involvement of the tibia in the same patient (lateral view).

933

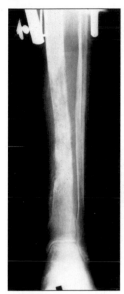

934

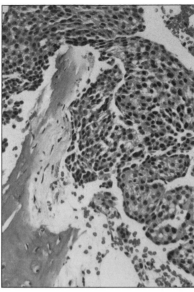

935

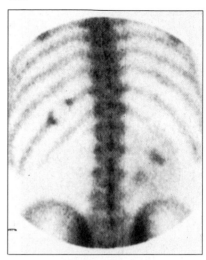

935 Rapidly growing rib metastases.

933 Three months later, where there has been rapid extension despite local radiotherapy to the area.

934 Histology of bone biopsy. There are clumps of an undifferentiated malignant tumour scattered within the bone. The appearances are in accordance with a primary in the bladder. *(H&E × 160)*

Local recurrence of tumours

Tumours can recur very rapidly and frequent cystoscopic examinations are obligatory, especially in the early stages and up to 5 years or longer.

936

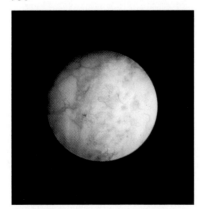

937

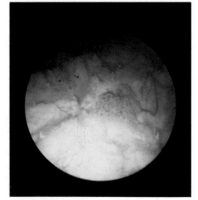

938

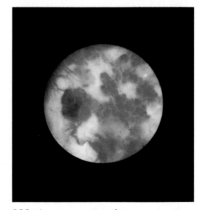

936 Early superficial recurrence of T2 tumour.

937 Sessile, almost confluent, recurrent T2 tumour.

938 A more extensive recurrence with a superficial haemorrhage in one of the tumours, T2 or T3a.

939

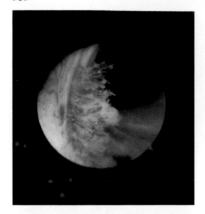

940

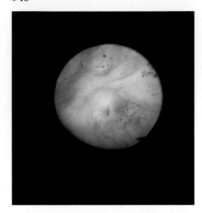

941

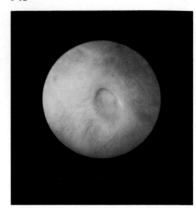

942

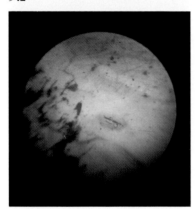

943

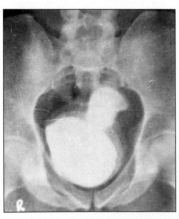

939 A recurrence of a T2 tumour in the prostatic cavity, a transurethral prostatic resection having been performed at the same time as the tumour resection.

When the tumour involves an orifice, the orifice should be completely ignored at the time of the initial resection because not only is it often never seen, but it will invariably re-epithelialise. It is much more important to be certain that the tumour is completely resected.

940 Orifice in the middle of scar tissue.

941 A similar orifice flattened and rigid, but not obstructed.

942 Even when there is deep excavation of an orifice at the time of the tumour resection, regrowth of epithelium will recur although the orifice may be gaping and will probably reflux; a small price if the tumour is controlled.

Occasionally a tumour can start in a diverticulum.

943 A filling defect and an irregular external wall of a diverticulum caused by an extensive tumour. Often these tumours can be visualised through an endoscope introduced through the mouth of the diverticulum. Ultrasound may help to delineate the tumour (see **924**).

Adenocarcinoma of the bladder

Adenocarcinoma of the bladder is rare and usually arises from the dome of the bladder. Sometimes it is palpable as a suprapubic mass.

944

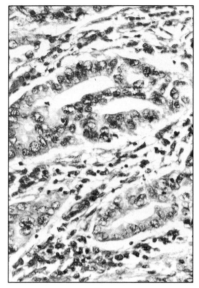

945

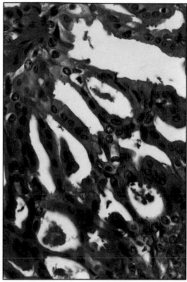

944 Histology of adenocarcinoma. This invasive tumour is composed of malignant cells making well-formed glandular structures. These tumours are rare and are particularly associated with urachal remnants and cystitis gland-ularis. *(H&E × 256)*

945 Glandular metaplasia may sometimes be seen in transitional cell carcinoma. It must be distinguished from an adenocarcinoma. This section shows gland-like spaces in a tumour which is basically transitional cell in type. *(H&E × 256)*

Squamous carcinoma of the bladder

The transitional cell lining of the blad-der easily undergoes squamous meta-plasia, and many transitional cell tu-mours show squamous metaplasia in some part of the tumour. However, the diagnosis of squamous carcinoma of the bladder should only be made when the whole of the tumour is composed of squamous cells. The endoscopic and IVU appearances are indisting-uishable from the advanced T3a, T3b, or T4 transitional cell carcinoma; the diagnosis is made by the pathologist.

946

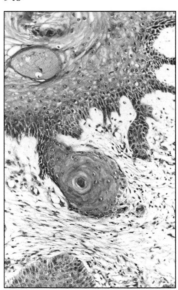

947

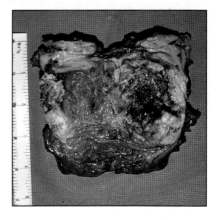

946 Histology of squamous cell carcinoma. This invasive tumour is composed predominantly of cells resembling the prickle cell layer of skin. It is forming keratin and there is a 'keratin pearl' in the middle of the field. These tumours are particularly associated with stones, diverticula, and bilharzia. *(H&E × 64)*

947 Cystectomy specimen of the bladder almost totally destroyed by a squamous cell carcinoma, which has covered almost the whole of the mucous membrane. It is sessile, invasive, and superficially ulcerated.

948

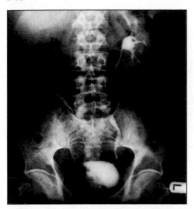

950

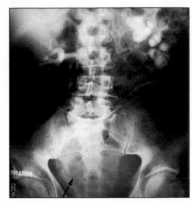

949

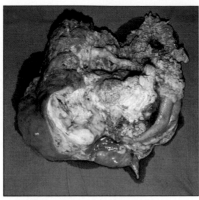

948 IVU of the same patient as 947. The tumour fills the right side of the bladder and completely obstructs the right ureter.

949 Cystectomy specimen showing total destruction of the bladder.

950 IVU showing a thin rim of dye on the right side of the bladder. This was a huge tumour, which not only involved the muscle layers, but almost completely filled the cavity of the bladder.

Industrial causes of bladder cancer

Industrial chemicals that have been accepted as a cause of bladder tumours are as follows and apply to people who work in a building in which any of the substances are produced or used for commercial purposes.

1 1-naphythlamine, previously known as alpha-naphythlamine.
2 2-naphythlamine, previously known as beta-naphythlamine.
3 Diphenyl substituted by one nitro or primary amino group.
4 Any of the substances mentioned in point 3 if a further ring is substituted by halogens, or a methyl, or methoxy group.
5 The salts of any of the substances mentioned in points 1–4.
6 Auramine or magenta. This applies to their manufacture and their use.

It is now thought that the toxicity of 1-naphthylamine is due to the presence of 2-napthylamine as an impurity. Two antioxidants N-phenyl-2-naphylamine (PBN) and N-phenyl-1-naphylamine (PAN) have also been incriminated as causes of industrial occupational bladder cancer and in both these compounds their contamination with 2-naphylamine may be the basic cause of this toxicity.

The only new compound to be added to the 1983 Prescribed Diseases List is 4,4'-methylenebis (2-chloroaniline) MBOCA. This product is widely used in the plastic industry and is undoubtedly carcinogenic in experimental animals. There is evidence that it may also be carcinogenic in man.

Chemical compounds
Chemical compounds have also been known to produce bladder cancer, and the two most important are:

● Phenacetin.
● Cyclophosphamide.

951–954 Chemicals involved in industrial bladder cancer. Clinicians caring for patients with urothelial tumours must always be aware of the possible association with industrial chemicals, or even drugs.

Predisposed occupations

For practical purposes, the following occupations should be especially noted:

- Factories manufacturing dyestuffs or pigments.
- Factories engaged in textile printing.
- Factories producing fine chemicals for laboratory use.
- Rubber or electric cable factories.
- Retort houses of gas works.
- Rat catchers who use antu, which contains 1-naphythlamine.
- Laboratory technicians who use the chemicals for routine testing.
- Workers in patent fuel manufacture.
- Sewage and water testing.

There is also evidence of an increased relative risk of bladder cancer in leather workers, hairdressers, machine tooling, driving and diesel exhaust exposure, and in aluminium refining.

Work with chemicals in the rubber or cable industry or any gasworks

On a more individual patient approach, each patient should be asked if they have ever worked with chemicals in the rubber or cable industry or any gas works and it must be remembered that there is a marked latent period, which can vary from 25–45 years between the exposure and the development of industrial cancer.

The tumour is first suspected when abnormal cells are found in the urine, and these are diagnosed by microscopy. The carcinoma may later spread to involve the uterus and vagina. Morphologically these tumours often start as carcinoma *in situ* in the bladder and tend to infiltrate the bladder wall and metastasise early.

951
952
953
954

Aniline
4 Aminodiphenyl
Diphenylamine
1- Naphthylamine
2- Naphthylamine
Benzidine
Dichlorbenzidine
Orthotoluidine
Auramine
Magenta

Locally extensive tumours

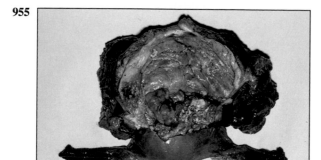

955 Cystectomy specimen of carcinoma of the bladder which has involved the body of the uterus. It was a squamous carcinoma starting in the fundus which had invaded in the uterus and the vagina.

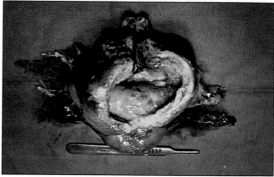

956 Cystectomy specimen of carcinoma invading urethra and vagina. Another squamous tumour which began at the base of the bladder and eventually ulcerated through the proximal urethra into the vagina.

Unusual tumours

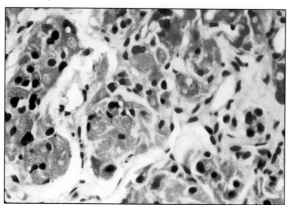

957 Phaeochromocystoma (nonchromaffin paraganglionoma of the bladder). The tumour is composed of nests of large cells with slightly granular cytoplasm. The nuclei are relatively small and usually centrally placed. Neurosecretory granules are present ultrastructurally. They are commonly present beneath the epithelium in or near the trigone, probably arising from nests of persistent paraganglion tissue. Behaviour is usually that of a benign tumour but metastasis has been recorded. *(H&E × 256)*

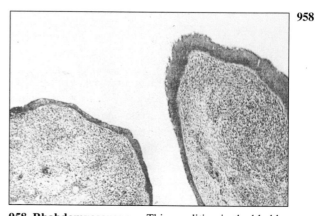

958 Rhabdomyosarcoma. This condition in the bladder occurs as embryonal or adult types. The type illustrated here occurs as a polypoid mass, which is often oedematous and likened in appearance to a bunch of grapes (sarcoma botryoides). The polyps are covered with transitional epithelium. In the underlying tissue is an infiltrate of small malignant cells, which can be mistaken for inflammation. *(H&E × 256)*

959

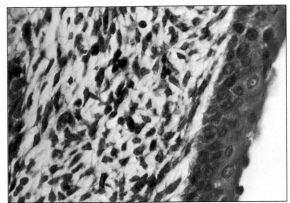

959 Rhabdomyosarcoma. Higher magnification of **958**, showing the oedematous stroma containing spindly cells. *(H&E × 256)*

960

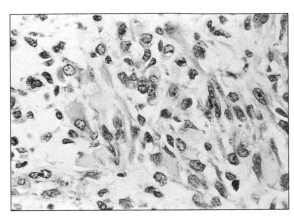

960 Rhabdomyosarcoma. Higher magnification of **958** showing strap-like cells. In the cytoplasm of some there are cross striations. *(H&E × 256)*

961

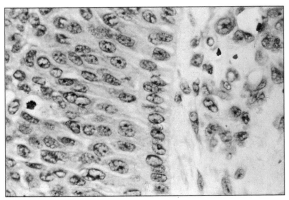

961 Carcinosarcoma. This is a biphasic tumour. On the left side of the field is malignant epithelium (carcinoma), and on the right are malignant cells growing in a sarcomatous pattern. It is probable that the tumour is basically a transitional cell carcinoma and that the 'sarcoma' is an unusual growth pattern of this tumour. *(H&E × 256)*

962

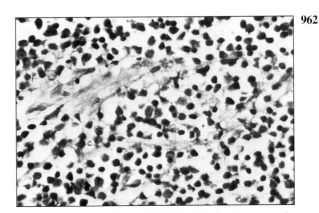

962 Malignant lymphoma. This may be primary or part of a systemic lymphoma. The tumour is composed of sheets of lymphoid cells. This lymphoma has the appearances of lymphosarcoma. It is important to distinguish it from reactive lymphoid tissue. *(H&E × 256)*

963

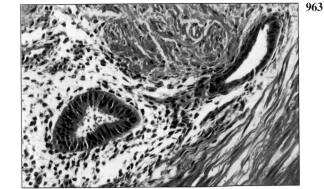

963 Endometriosis may form a tumour-like mass in the wall of the bladder. Histology shows two essential elements for diagnosis. First there are endometrium-type glands: second there are endometrial stromal cells around them. The bladder muscle is outside this. *(H&E × 64)*

964

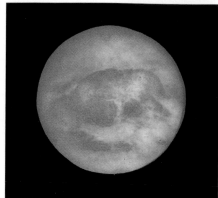

Amyloid

964 Endoscopy reveals a solid vascular mass simulating a carcinoma and only distinguishable on histology from a neoplasm.

965 Section through a tumour-like mass of amyloid in the bladder. It shows a mass of reddish material in the lamina propria covered by transitional epithelium. *(Sirius red × 64)*

966 Amyloid is a term applied to a number of abnormal fibrillary proteins, a characteristic of which is that they stain with dyes like Sirius red (or Congo red) and subsequently, when viewed with crossed polaroids, are birefringent and dichroic. This section shows amyloid giving a green colour, while the collagen (which is also birefringent) is yellow. *(Sirius red: crossed polaroids × 160)*

965

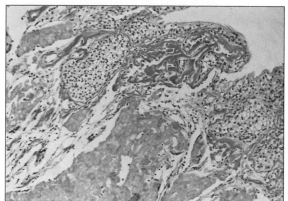

966

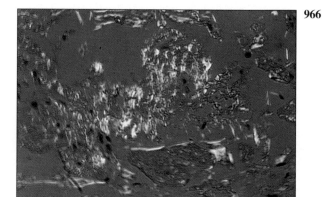

967

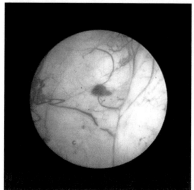

967 Bladder haemangioma. Small vascular malformations are occasionally seen in the bladder. The lesion shown here as a mucosal bluish mass proved entirely benign on histology.

968

968 Bladder haemangioma. A haemangioma is a vascular malformation composed of thin-walled vascular channels lined with endothelium and filled with blood. In this section the attentuated epithelium (at the top) covers blood-filled channels of various sizes. *(H&E × 160)*

9 Diseases of the prostate

Diseases of the prostate and bladder neck, together with urethral stricture (see Chapter 10) are responsible for the main causes of urinary outflow obstruction in the male.

Benign prostatic hypertrophy and carcinoma of the prostate are dealt with in two separate sections in this chapter.

Benign prostatic hypertrophy and bladder-neck obstruction

Benign enlargement of the prostate is a complex pathological process that tends to arise in relation to the central group of prostatic glands and may lead to urethral compression. However, the changes may be confined to the bladder-neck region. Either type of process may lead to outflow obstruction. The classic presentation of prostatism – hesitancy in starting micturition, a poor urinary stream, and post-micturition dribbling is often associated with nocturia. Occasionally haematuria and urgency may occur, and there is dysuria when urinary tract infection supervenes. The presence of residual urine encourages this complication.

969

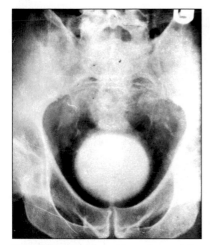

969 The post-micturition phase of the IVU shows residual urine and bladder wall thickening.

970

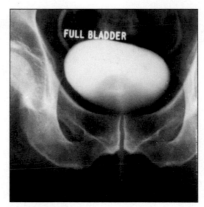

970 Prostatic hypertrophy may be observed by the presence of a prostatic impression in the bladder base, but this is an unreliable sign for assessing prostatic size.

971

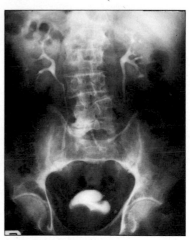

971 When haematuria is a presenting symptom, it must not be forgotten that bladder tumours do coexist; the filling defects of both a bladder tumour and benign prostatic hypertrophy are seen in this bladder film, underlying the need for cystoscopy in every case of prostatic pathology.

972

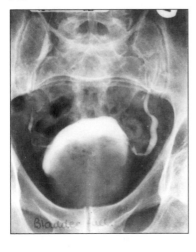

973

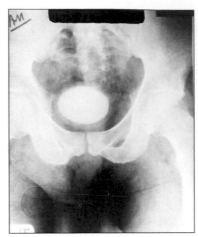

972 A gross prostatic impression with ureteric hooking.

973 Bladder-neck obstruction. In obstruction by the bladder neck alone, the bladder is thickened and spherical with no basal impression.

Ultrasound

974

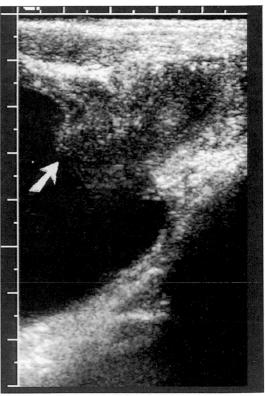

974 Typical scan of patient with benign prostatic hyperplasia showing a rounded intact capsule and a homogenous parenchymal echo pattern.

975

975 Sagittal transrectal ultrasound in a patient with benign prostatic hyperplasia. The adenoma is predominantly echo-poor and is invaginating the bladder base (arrow).

976

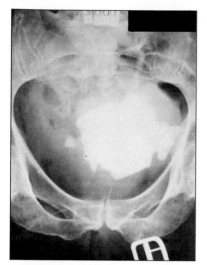

976 Calculi may form as a result of in-complete bladder emptying.

977

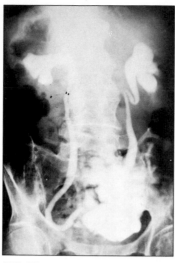

977 The obstructed upper tracts with ureteric hooking, particularly marked on the left side, are seen in this patient with a large irregular bladder calculus.

978

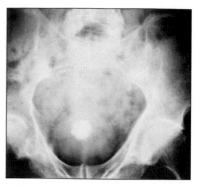

978 Phosphatic calculi are frequently smooth and ovoid in shape.

979

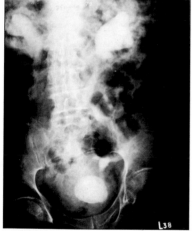

979 Upper tract dilatation is shown in this patient with a bladder calculus.

980

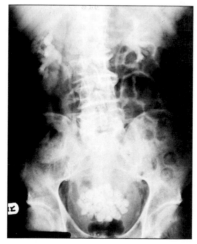

980 There may be multiple bladder calculi.

981

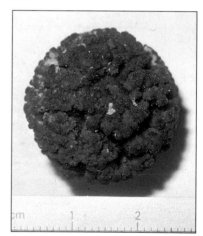

981 An oxalate calculus. The irregular surface is covered with blood pigments.

982

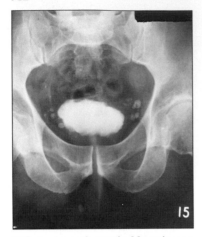

982 An irregular vesical base is seen in this patient with uric acid stones. The calculi are radiolucent.

983

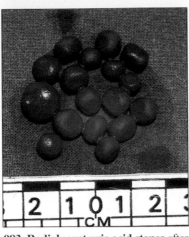

983 Radiolucent uric acid stones after removal, surrounded by blood pigment.

984

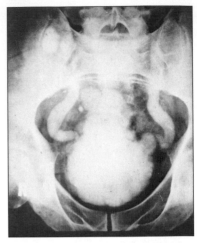

984 Classic bilateral ureteric hold-up demonstrating the 'fish-hook' deformity.

985

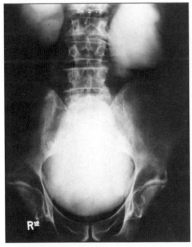

985 There may be progression to bilateral hydronephrosis with chronic retention and obstruction.

986

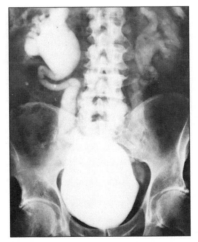

986 Reflux may also occur as seen here on the right side.

987

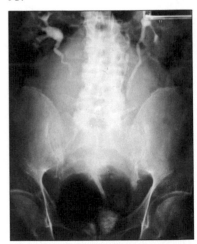

987 Chronic retention (here associated with gross prostatic calcification) may not affect the upper tracts, which here are seen to be normal.

988

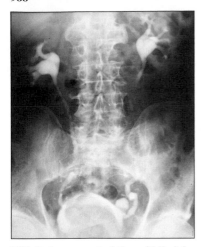

988 Enlargement of the middle lobe may be demonstrated as an intravesical filling defect. Note the normal upper tracts. It may be differentiated from clot by its smooth outline.

989

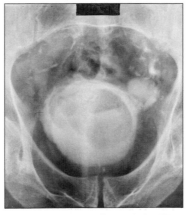

989 The vesical film of the IVU shows the middle lobe filling defect apparently unattached to the bladder base. A small left-sided diverticulum is also present.

990

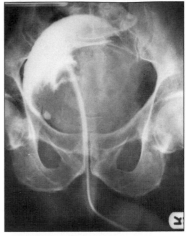

990 Clot in the bladder shows two appearances of a patchy irregular defect not unlike a tumour.

991

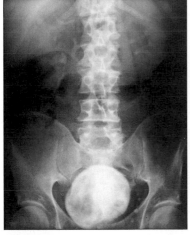

991 Full bladder also containing clot.

992

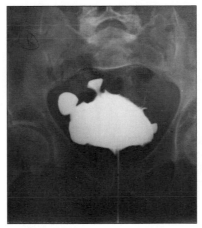

992 Multiple small diverticula may result from obstruction.

993

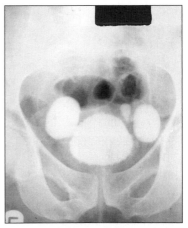

993 Two larger diverticula on either side of the bladder.

994

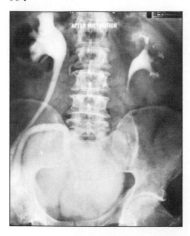

995

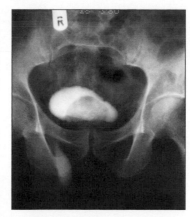

994 In this patient with a very large right-sided diverticulum the tortuous course of the right ureter is easily seen.

995 The bladder may also enter hernial sacs as a pseudodiverticulum.

996

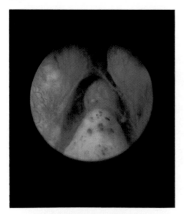

996 Retention of urine may be acute and painful or chronic and painless. The distended bladder is easily visible in the abdomen of this patient with chronic retention.

Endoscopy

997

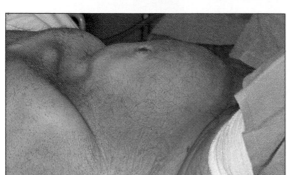

998

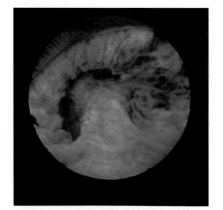

999

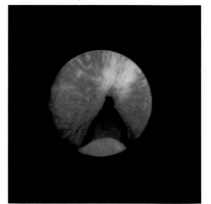

997 Small pigmented lesions are frequently seen on the urethral crest.

998 Endoscopy is essential to assess prostatic obstruction and must always precede surgery. The verumontanum marking the prostatic apex is shown.

999 Moving through the prostatic urethra the lateral lobes are seen projecting in over the verumontanum.

1000

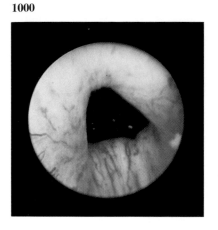

1001

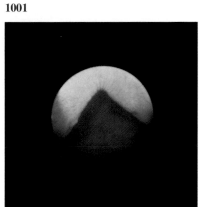

1000 At the internal meatus, a middle lobe is shown between the inverted V of the lateral lobes.

1001 In the upper portion of the urethra at the bladder neck, early lateral lobe enlargement is shown.

1002

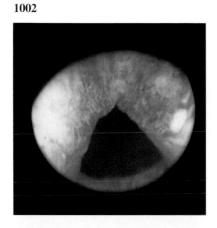

1003

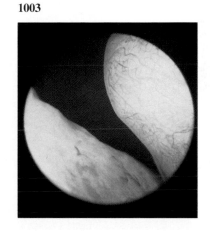

1002 Increasing lateral lobe enlargement at the bladder neck.

1003 A narrow anterior angle with asymmetrical enlargement of the lateral lobes.

1004

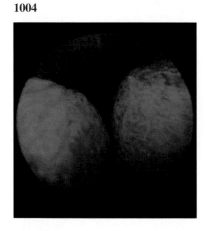

1005

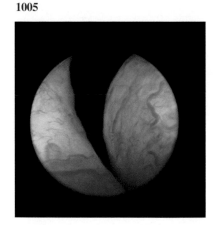

1004 Bilateral symmetrical lateral lobe enlargement.

1005 Unilateral enlargement of the left lobe.

1006

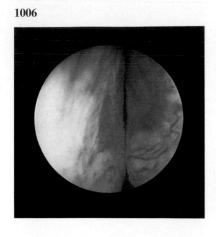

1007

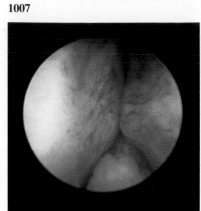

1006 The enlarged lobes meet in the mid-line.

1007 In the distal portion of the prostatic urethra the verumontanum appears between the enlarged lateral lobes.

1008

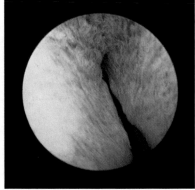

1009

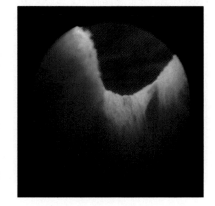

1008 Inflammatory changes may be seen with injection of the vessels lying on the surface of the lateral lobes.

1009 Inflammatory changes at the bladder neck.

1010

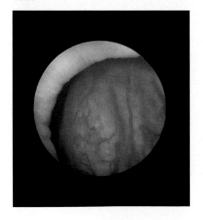

1011

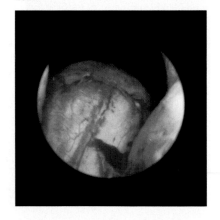

1010 An enlarged and inflamed middle lobe.

1011 A very large middle lobe.

1012

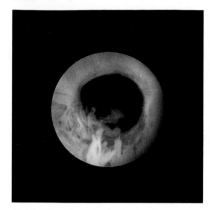

1013

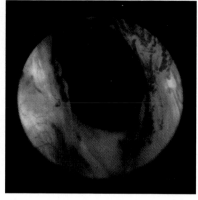

1014

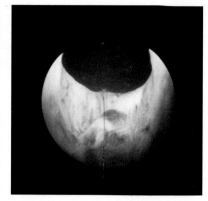

1012 The obstruction may be caused by sclerosis of the bladder-neck tissues.

1013 Fibrosis may be marked in this process.

1014 The crescentic appearance of the early obstructing bladder neck.

1015, 1016 Bladder-neck obstruction with early lateral lobe enlargement seen by rigid (**1015**) and flexible (**1016**) cystoscopy.

1015

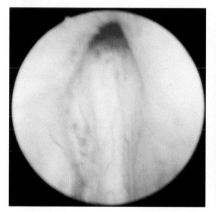

1016

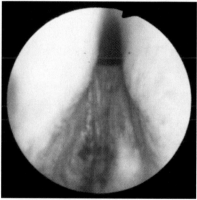

1017

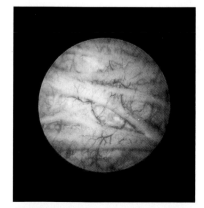

1018

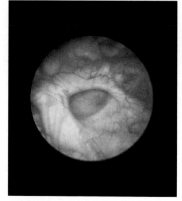

1019

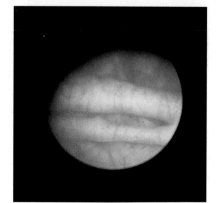

1017 The bladder responds to outflow obstruction by hypertrophy. Classic 'ribbing' of the thickened muscle is seen (i.e. trabeculation).

1018 Increased trabeculation with early sacculation. This may advance to diverticulum formation.

1019 Coarse trabeculation.

1020

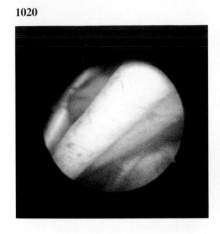

1021

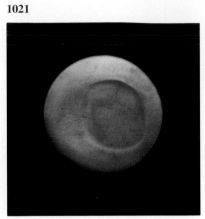

1020 Very coarse trabeculation. Note the clot lying between the trabeculae.

1021 A shallow diverticulum.

1022

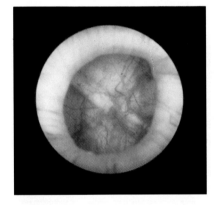

1023

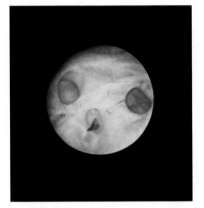

1022 The mouth of a large diverticulum.

1023 Multiple diverticula.

1024

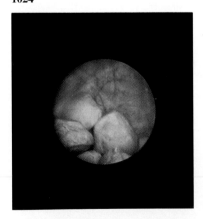

1025

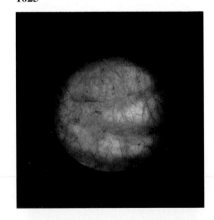

1024 Calculi in a trabeculated bladder.

1025 Urinary tract infection, a consequence of residual urine and superadded infection produces cystitis and results in an infected trabeculated bladder. Here there is inflamed trabeculated bladder wall.

1026

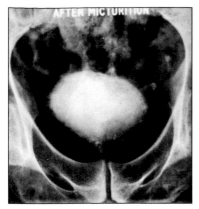

1027

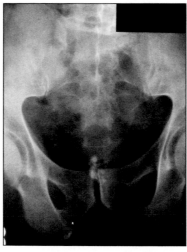

1028

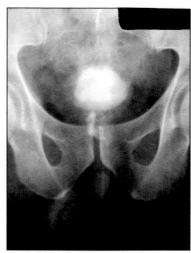

1026 Prostatic calcification can occur either with or without infection. Chronic bacterial prostatitis is usually accompanied by calculus formation in the prostate. Here there is considerable residual urine with small prostatic calculi beneath the bladder base. Phleboliths (calcification in pelvic veins) are also present.

1027 A large prostatic calculus.

1028 Post-micturition film showing residual urine in this patient.

1029

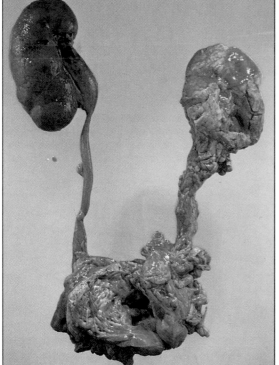

1030

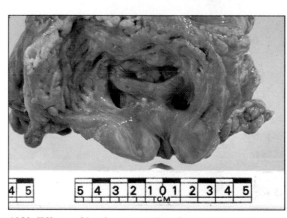

1030 Effects of benign prostatic enlargement. A close-up of the bladder of the specimen seen in **1029** showing the enlarged prostate with the thick-walled bladder distorted by muscle bands and diverticula.

1029 Effects of benign prostatic enlargement. A postmortem specimen showing an enlarged prostate, which has produced a trabecular bladder with multiple diverticula. There is bilateral hydroureter and hydronephrosis.

1031

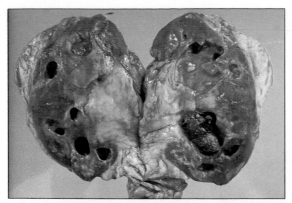

1031 Effects of benign prostatic enlargement. A close-up of the bisected left kidney seen in **1029** showing the hydro-ureter, hydronephrosis, and a stone in the pelvis at the lower pole.

1032

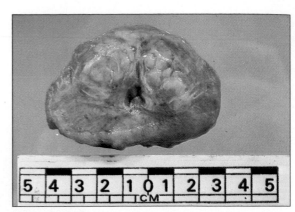

1032 Benign prostatic enlargement. A transverse section through the nodular enlarged prostate seen in **1029**. In this condition the enlargement affects the periurethral portion of the prostate (median and lateral lobes).

1033

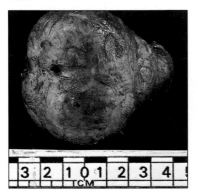

1033 Benign prostatic enlargement. A surgical specimen of a nodular enlarged prostate.

1034

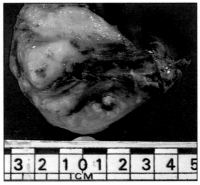

1034 Benign prostatic enlargement. Sagittal section through the specimen seen in **1033** .

1035

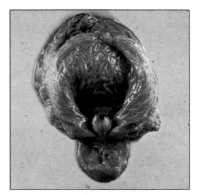

1035 Benign prostatic enlargement. Postmortem specimen of bladder and prostate showing median lobe enlargement and trabeculation of the bladder.

1036

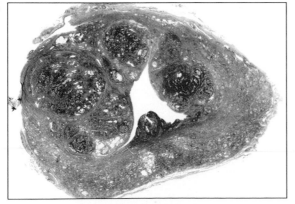

1037

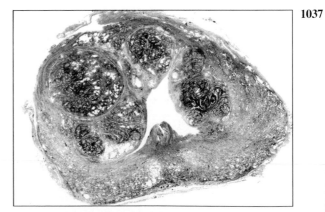

1036, 1037 Benign enlargement of the prostate is caused by hyperplasia and/or hypertrophy of tissues normally found in the prostate. The major elements are glandular, muscular, and fibrous tissue. Enlargement usually shows a mixture of these elements though one or other can predominate. Median lobe enlargement is often solid, with fibrous and muscular tissue predominating. Nodules in the lateral lobes usually have a large glandular component. These two sections of a postmortem specimen of prostate show the nodular enlargement affecting large areas of the gland. The trichrome picks up the fibrous tissue (stained green). (*Natural size: H&E and trichrome*)

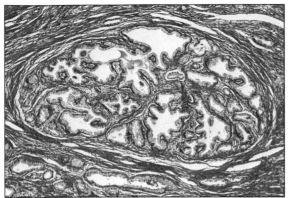

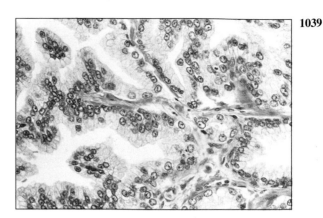

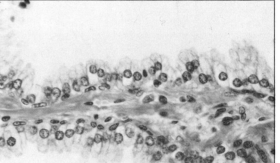

1038 Adenomyomatous hyperplasia. A small nodule composed of glands and bands of fibrous tissue, and muscle is arranged around it. *(H&E × 26)*

1039 Adenomyomatous hyperplasia. Part of a nodule composed of hyperplastic glands showing papillary infolding of the tall columnar epithelium. There is little connective tissue between the glands. *(H&E × 160)*

1040 Adenomyomatous hyperplasia. Higher magnification to show the epithelium of hyperplastic glands. There is a two-layered arrangement with tall columnar epithelium lining the lumen of the gland and a basal layer of cells lying beneath them. *(H&E × 256)*

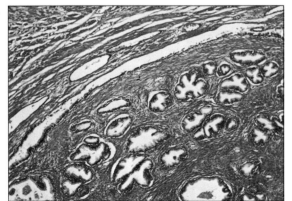

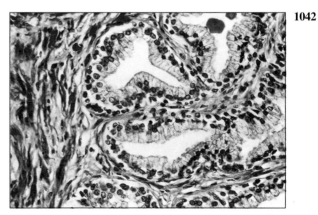

1041 Fibroadenomatous hyperplasia. Part of the edge of a nodule that shows glandular hyperplasia, but in which there is a much more prominent connective tissue component. This is predominantly fibrous. *(H&E × 26)*

1042 Fibroadenomatous hyperplasia. Higher magnification to show glands with smooth muscle fibres (red) and (green). *(Trichrome × 160)*

1043

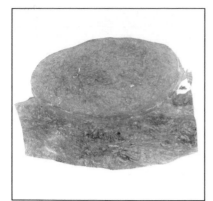

1044

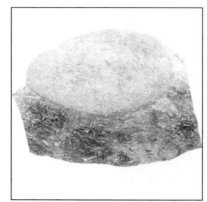

1043, 1044 Fibromyomatous nodule. This solid type of nodule lacks a glandular element and is composed of varying proportions of muscle and fibrous tissue. Some small subepithelial nodules close to the urethra are composed of loose fibrovascular connective tissue with little muscle: such nodules are often called stromal nodules. *(Natural size: H&E and trichrome)*

1045

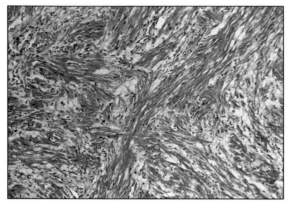

1045 Fibromyomatous nodule. A solid nodule composed of smooth muscle and fibrous tissue. *(H&E × 64)*

1046

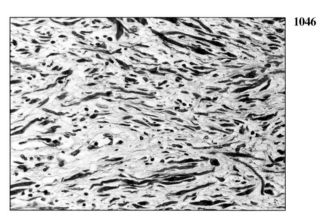

1046 Fibromyomatous nodule. Similar area stained to show fibrous tissue (green) and smooth muscle cells (red). *(Trichrome × 160)*

1047 Prostate: infarct with squamous metaplasia. Occasionally prostatic nodules infarct. Often adjacent epithelium then undergoes a change that makes it look like squamous epithelium. This section shows an area of infarction on the right side of the field. There is an inflammatory reaction at the junction of the dead and the viable tissue. The epithelium shows 'squamous metaplasia'. *(H&E × 64)*

1047

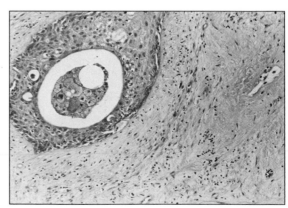

Carcinoma of the prostate

In contrast to benign hypertrophy, carcinoma of the prostate usually arises in relation to the peripheral group of prostatic glands. Nevertheless, infiltration of the gland by the malignant process will produce outflow obstruction with all the radiological appearances shown in the benign disease.

The serum prostatic specific antigen (PSA) (normal 0–4 µg/ litre) test has been introduced and is being used increasingly in patients with carcinoma of the prostate. Discussion still continues as to whether it should be used widely as a screening test. While high values above 25 µg/litre frequently indicate disseminated disease, large benign glands can produce false positive elevations and high levels up to 100 µg/litre can occur in patients with localised prostatic carcinoma.

TNM clinical classification

T (primary tumour)

TX Primary tumour cannot be assessed.
T0 No evidence of primary tumour.
T1 Clinically inapparent tumour not palpable or visible by imaging.
  T1a Tumour incidental finding in 5% or less of tissue resected.
  T1b Tumour incidental finding in more than 5% of tissue resected.
  T1c Tumour identified by needle biopsy (e.g. because of elevated PSA).
T2 Tumour confirmed within prostate (*i).
  T2a Tumour involves 50% of a lobe or less.
  T2b Tumour involves more than 50% of a lobe, but not both lobes.
  T2c Tumour involves both lobes.

T3 Tumour extends through prostate capsule (*ii).
  T3a Unilateral extracapsular extension.
  T3b Bilateral extracapsular extension.
  T3c Tumour invades seminal vesicle(s).
T4 Tumour is fixed or invades adjacent structures other than seminal vesicles.
  T4a Tumour invades any of the following: bladder neck, external sphincter, rectum.
  T4b Tumour invades levator muscle and/or is fixed to pelvic wall.

* Notes:
i. Tumour found in one or both lobes by needle biopsy, but not palpable or visible by imaging is classified as T1c.
ii. Invasion into the prostatic apex or into (but not beyond) the prostatic capsule is not classified as T3, but as T2.

N (regional lymph nodes)

N1 Single node < than 2 cm.
N2 Single node > than 2–5 cm or multiple < than 5 cm.
N3 > than 5 cm.

M (distant metastasis)

MX Presence of distant metastasis can not be assessed.
M0 No distant metastasis.
M1 Distant metastasis.
  M1a Nonregional lymph node(s).
  M1b Bone(s).
  M1c Other site(s).

UICC (TNM) classification as applied to prostatic tumours

Tx Incidental carcinoma in operative specimen (i.e. no pre-operative evidence of carcinoma or where the carcinoma was previously unsuspected). This will be linked with a P category in the operative specimen.

T1 Intracapsular malignancy involving less than 50% total volume of prostate in an otherwise normal or hypertrophied gland – the nodule.

T2 Intracapsular malignancy involving more than 50% of the volume of an otherwise normal or hypertrophic gland.

T3 Malignancy extending beyond the capsule into the paraprostatic tissue. This includes cases with involvement of seminal vesicle, ulceration in the posterior urethra, or invasion of the bladder neck.

T4 Malignancy fixed to the pelvic wall and/or involvement of rectum and/or bladder beyond the bladder neck.

To No evidence of primary growth, but clinical diagnosis of metastatic prostatic carcinoma made. (Will be linked with N2 or M1 category).

Tis Pre-invasive carcinoma (carcinoma *in situ*).

Px Pathologist is not able to give extent of the tumour, but did have malignant tissue available for examination – as found in routine TURP.

P1 Malignant intracapsular nodule occupying less than 50% volume of the whole prostate.

P2 Malignant change involving more than 50% volume of the prostate.

P3 Involvement of capsule or incomplete removal of malignancy.

G (histopathological grading)

G1 High degree of differentiation.

G2 Medium degree of differentiation or undifferentiated.

G3 Low degree of differentiation or undifferentiated.

GX Grade cannot be assessed.

1048

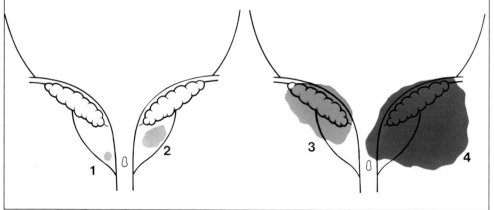

1048 Diagram of the clinical stages of carcinoma of prostate. Clinically the gland may feel and look benign and the diagnosis is only made from the histology of the resected specimen. Because this process often arises in the periphery of the gland, biopsy by the perineal or transrectal route of palpable nodules may be required to prove the diagnosis.

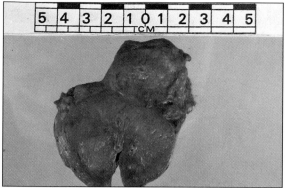

1049 Carcinoma of the prostate. Postmortem specimen of a prostate showing a nodule extending posteriorly outside the capsule. The nodule and much of the prostate showed adenocarcinoma. The patient died with multiple metastases.

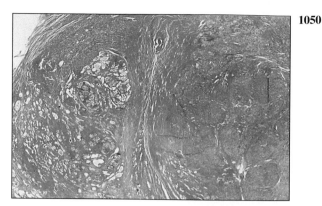

1050 Section of prostate from radical prostatectomy specimen showing large tumour nodule in right lobe with smaller peripheral nodule in left lobe. *(H&E)*

Ultrasound

Ultrasound is the most effective modality for assessment of prostate tumours.

1051 Colour Doppler transverse axial transrectal ultrasound in a patient with a T1 prostate cancer. There is an echo-poor area in the left peripheral zone of the gland associated with localised increased blood flow.

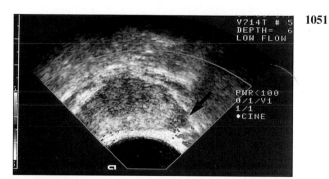

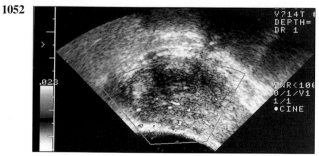

1052 Transverse axial colour Doppler transrectal ultrasound in a patient with a T2 prostate cancer. There is an irregular echo-poor area involving the peripheral and central parts of the prostate associated with increased blood flow. The capsule of the gland is intact.

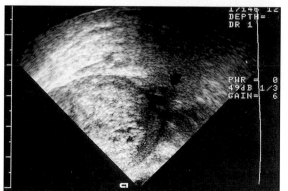

1053 Transverse axial transrectal ultrasound in a patient with T3 prostate cancer. An echo-poor area in the left peripheral zone of the prostate is extending into the central part of the gland and beyond the capsule of the gland (arrow).

233

1054

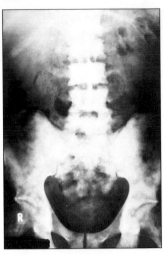

1055

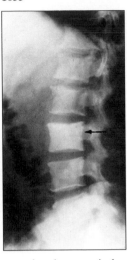

1056

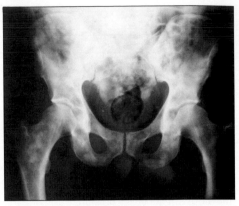

1056 The pelvic bones are often involved in carcinoma of the prostate.

1054 Carcinoma of the prostate frequently spreads to bone, particularly the lumbar spine, via the valveless veins communicating between the periprostatic and perivertebral plexuses. Osteosclerotic metastases are usually diffuse and occur in 80% of such patients.

1055 A lateral view of the lumbar spine shows a sclerotic body of the third lumbar vertebra. A raised prostatic specific antigen (PSA) invariably accompanies these bone changes.

1057

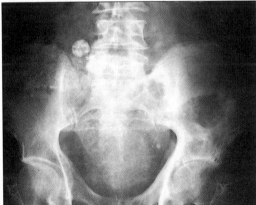

1058

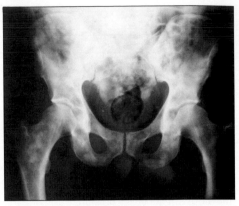

1059

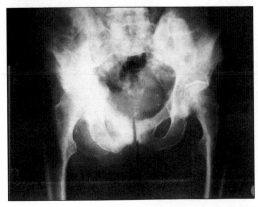

1057 Paget's disease for comparison shows coarse bony trabeculae with expansion of the bone. These changes are often unilateral as is seen here, with an essentially normal right ilium.

1058 Gross involvement of the whole pelvis, especially the right ischiopubic and iliopubic rami. There is sclerosis, but little enlargement.

1059 The rare destructive form of bony metastases.

1060

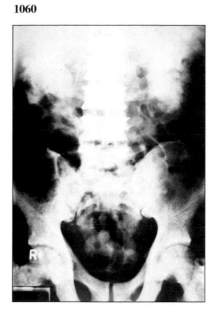

1061

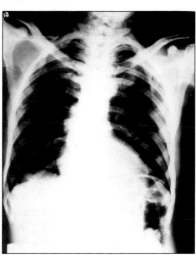

1060 IVU showing gross bilateral hydronephrosis. There is marked density of the lumbar spine.

1061 Widespread metastases in the ribs.

1062

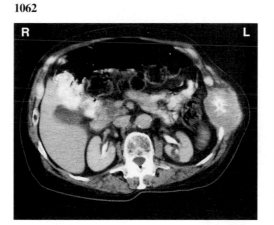

1063

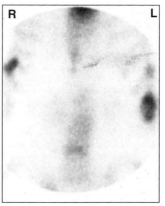

1062, 1063 Bony metastases can sometimes be very localised as in **1062** (bone scan showing large metastasis in the lower left rib cage) and **1063** (large metastasis in a lower left rib which presented as a palpable mass).

1064 Soft tissue metastases. Bilateral hilar lymphadenopathy with nodules through both lung fields. This patient had a negative bone scan, but a PSA level of 1600 μg/litre.

1064

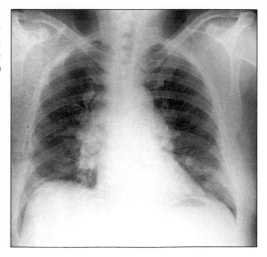

1065

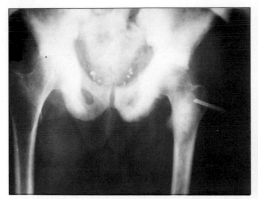

**1065 Both the pelvis and left femur are involved
with a pathological fracture of the femoral neck.**

1066

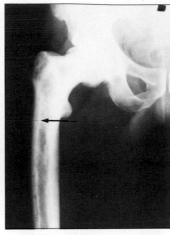

1066 Paget's disease of the femur
showing bone expansion and bow-
ing with a fracture of the lateral
border.

1067

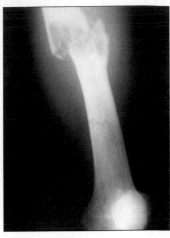

**1067 Pathological fracture of
femoral shaft.**

Bone scanning by radioisotope techniques

Bone scintigraphy by ^{99M} technetium (^{99M} Tc)
allows imaging of bony metastases shown by
the increased uptake in the new bone provoked
by the underlying metastases.

1068 A bone scan, which is effectively a superscan,
demonstrates widespread metastases involving
almost the whole of the bony skeleton.

1068

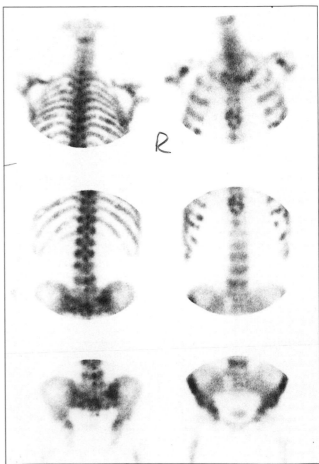

Endoscopy

1069, 1070 Endoscopy shows the 'shaggy' irregular appearance of the malignant disease process involving the lateral lobes and ulcerating the urethral surface.

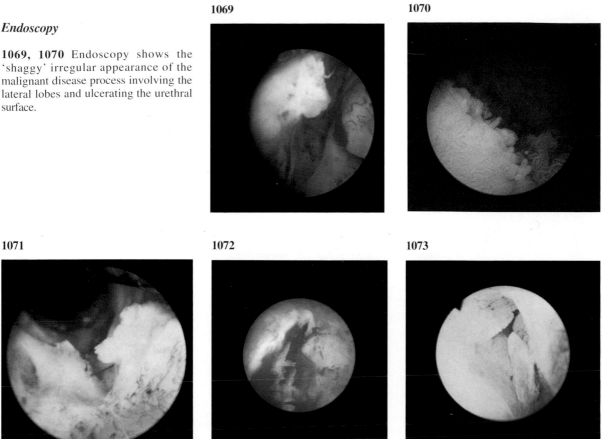

1069

1070

1071

1072

1073

1071, 1072, 1073 The endoscopic appearance may resemble that of benign disease in the early stages as the disease process begins peripherally and accompanying benign processes may have involved the periurethral tissues.

Grading of prostatic adenocarcinoma

Many methods have been evolved for the grading of prostatic adenocarcinoma. Grading of a tumour involves a histological assessment of degree of differentiation. This grading is often used to predict behaviour and sometimes to guide treatment. The higher the grade of a tumour the less well it resembles its parent cells and the poorer its prognosis (for tumours of the same stage).

Many factors may be taken into account in a grading scheme. In prostatic adenocarcinoma gland formation, nuclear size, nuclear shape, nuclear atypia, mitotic count, nucleoli number and other factors have all been considered and many schemes have been evolved. In the UK, a simple grading scheme into well, moderately and poorly differentiated adenocarcinoma is most widely used

and is illustrated here. In the USA where radical prostatectomy is more commonly performed the Gleason system of grading is extensively used and is claimed to be a more valuable predictor. It is based on low power microscopy and assessment of histological patterns of tumour growth and infiltration. It does not depend on cytological features of individual cells. Five patterns are recognized:

1. Round glands, closely packed together, the tumour having a sharply demarcated margin (**1074**).

2. Less uniform glands, irregularly arranged, varying in size and shape. The margins are irregular and the tumour shows some infiltration (**1075**).

3. The glands may be single and show variation in size, shape and architecture. There may be some heaping up of epithelium and sometimes a cribriform arrangement. The tumour is infiltrative with ill-defined margins (**1076**).

4. The tumour is composed of sheets of cells often with an extensive clear cell pattern with pseudoluminal spaces. It is infiltrative with diffuse growth through stroma with ragged, infiltrative margins (**1077–1079**).

5. Anaplastic carcinoma growing in sheets or cords infiltrating through connective tissue and muscle. Glandular differentiation minimal or absent (**1080** and **1081**).

A predominant and secondary pattern is recognised for each tumour and points (1 to 5) are given for the two patterns. The points are added to give a total (2 to 10) and this is the Gleason score. Where only one pattern is recognised the points for the pattern are doubled to give the final score.

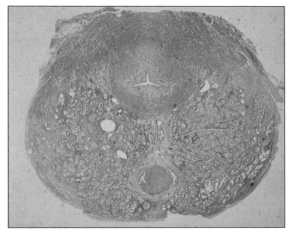

1074 A small well-circumscribed adenocarcinoma is present in the posterior lobe. The tumour has a sharply demarcated margin (whole prostrate, low magnification). (**Gleason 1**)

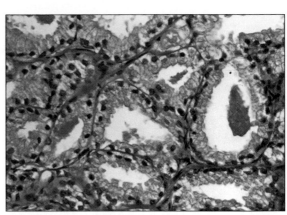

1075 Well-differentiated adenocarcinoma of the prostate. Part of a prostate nodule in which the glands are small and rounded, and lack myoepithelial cells. This is a well-differentiated adenocarcinoma. When such lesions are small, confined to the prostate, and do not show undifferentiated cells, the outlook is good and treatment is not normally indicated. (*H&E × 256*) (**Gleason 2**)

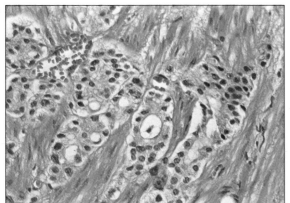

1076 Prostate: adenocarcinoma. A well-differentiated carcinoma composed of well-formed small glands which appear to be cutting across muscle. (*H&E × 256*) (**Gleason 3**)

1077

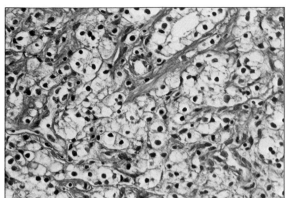

1077 Prostate: adenocarcinoma. Almost all carcinomas of the prostate are adenocarcinomas of varying degrees of differentiation. Other carcinomas (such as transitional cell and squamous cell) occur infrequently. Sarcomas are very rare. This section shows moderately differentiated adenocarcinoma composed of small acini crowded together. *(H&E × 160)* (**Gleason 4**)

1078

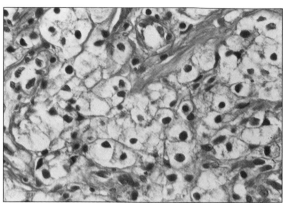

1078 Prostate adenocarcinoma. A higher magnification showing the nests of cells with clear cytoplasm and hyperchromatic, but not particularly large or pleomorphic nuclei. *(H&E × 256)* (**Gleason 4**)

1079

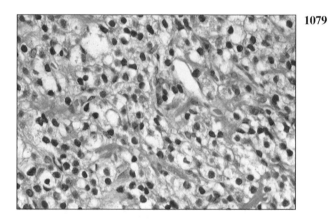

1079 Prostate: poorly differentiated adenocarcinoma. In this tumour, groups of tumour cells occupy most of the field, but only occasional gland-like forms are seen. *(H&E × 256)* (**Gleason 4**)

1080

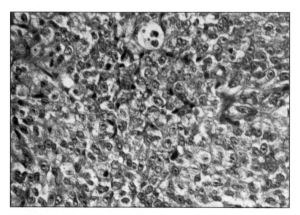

1080 Prostate: anaplastic carcinoma. This tumour shows no evidence of differentiation towards glandular or other epithelium. *(H&E × 256)* (**Gleason 5**)

1081

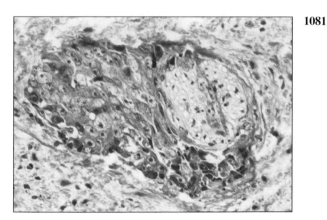

1081 Prostate: adenocarcinoma: perineural invasion. Adenocarcinoma may invade along tissue planes and is particularly likely to invade around nerves. The observation of perineural invasion may help in making the diagnosis of carcinoma in well-differentiated lesions. *(H&E × 160)* (**Gleason 5**)

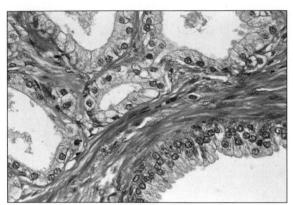

1082 Prostate: atypical hyperplasia. Sometimes a glandular proliferation shows cellular atypicality without evidence of invasion. The glands in the upper part of the field show some abnormal features, but carcinoma can not be diagnosed. The term 'atypical hyperplasia' is widely used for such appearances; the significance of these appearances is unclear. The gland in the bottom right corner is simply hyperplastic. *(H&E × 160)*

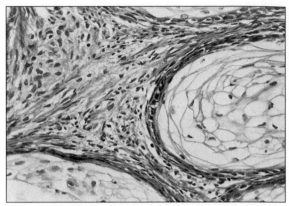

1083 Prostate: adenocarcinoma: oestrogen treatment. Oestrogen therapy for carcinoma often results in the development in the epithelium of large pale cells with small pyknotic nuclei. This appearance resembles stratified squamous epithelium and is called squamous metaplasia. *(H&E × 160)*

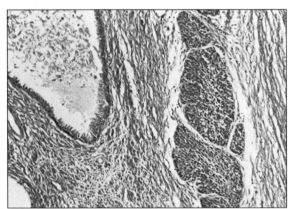

1084 Prostate: transitional cell carcinoma. Transitional cell carcinoma can arise in the prostatic ducts without tumour being present in the bladder of urethra. Such a tumour is seen here. There are normal prostatic glands on the left side of the picture while the solid clumps of epithelial cells have the appearances of a transitional cell carcinoma. These tumours do not respond to oestrogens and behave in a similar fashion to transitional cell carcinoma in the bladder. *(H&E × 64)*

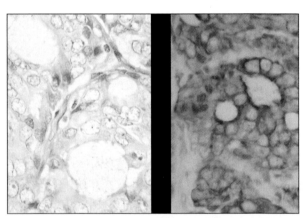

1085 Prostatic specific antigen. Sections from an enlarged lymph node in a 62-year-old man. The H&E section on the left shows an adenocarcinoma. On the right an indirect immunoperoxidase for PSA shows extensive staining in the cytoplasm of tumour cells, leading to a diagnosis of metastatic prostatic adenocarcinoma. *(H&E, indirect immunoperoxidase for PSA, × 160)*

10 Urethral inflammation, stricture, and tumours

Urethral disorders are principally inflammatory in origin. The male urethra is particularly prone to post-inflammatory stricture formation. Neoplastic lesions also occasionally arise in the urethra.

1086

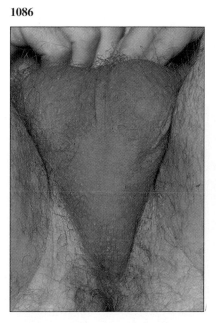

1087

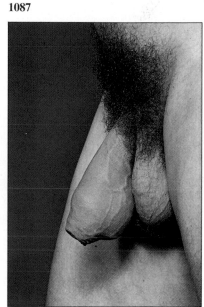

1086 Urethral inflammatory disease may arise in the periurethral glands causing perineal abscess.

1087 A paraurethral abscess secondary to gonorrhoea.

Urethritis caused by nonspecific urethritis or gonorrhoea presents with urethral discharge and dysuria. It may also be associated with urinary tract infections.

1088

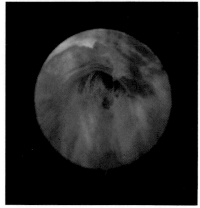

1089

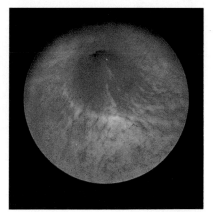

1088 Acute inflammation in the anterior urethra close to the glans.

1089 Mild inflammatory changes in the penile urethra.

1090

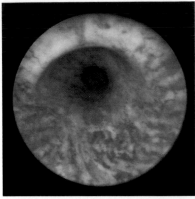

1091

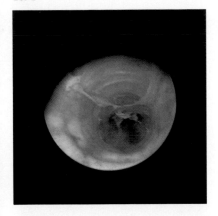

1090 Mild inflammation in the membranous urethra.

1091 Inflammation superimposed on a chronic stricture.

1092

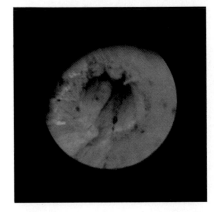

1093

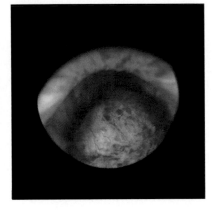

1092 Inflammatory changes in the region of the external sphincter.

1093 Acute inflammatory changes surrounding the verumontanum.

1094

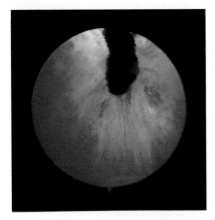

1094 Inflammation involving the prostate and prostatic urethra.

1095

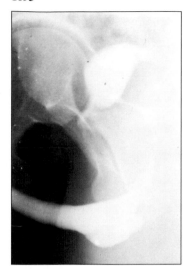

1096

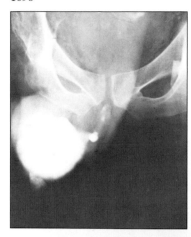

1095 Congenital urethral diverticula may be found and often present with urinary tract infection.

1096 Large urethral diverticulum.

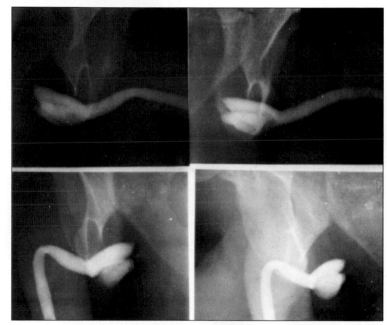

1097

1097 Ascending urethrography will demonstrate the diverticulum.

1098, 1099 Urethral calculi may be formed in diverticula as shown here or may impact in the urethra having formed higher in the urinary tract. Occasionally a urethral diverticulum forms after trauma.

1098

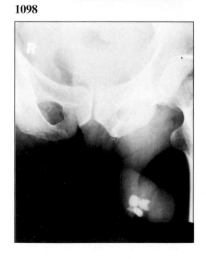

1099

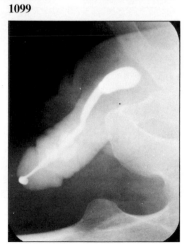

1100

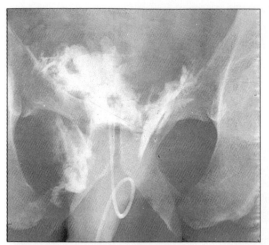

1100 Extravasation of contrast indicates urethral and bladder damage. Note the fractured pelvis.

1101

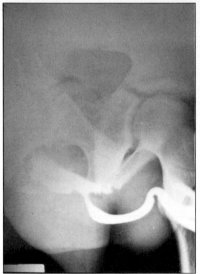

1102

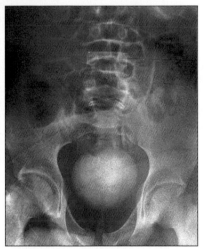

1101 Trauma to the membranous urethra often accompanies unstable pelvic fractures, when the perineal membrane becomes unstable and a shearing force is transmitted to the urethra. Bleeding per urethram strongly suggests this injury; ascending urethrography with water soluble contrast media provides the diagnosis.

1102 IVU showing elevation of bladder and medial deviation of lower ureter after urethral trauma. Note the fractured pelvis.

1104

Fistula

1103

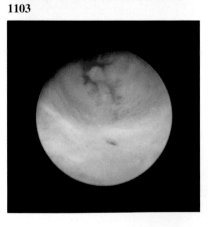

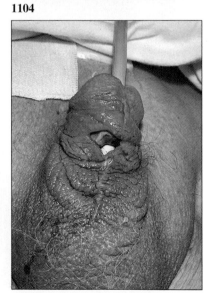

1103 Endoscopy will locate the site of a fistula in the rare situation when the urethra is involved in inflammatory or neoplastic disease. This fistula followed a severe urethral injury.

1104 Fistulae may also result from long-term catheterisation.

Urethral stricture

1105

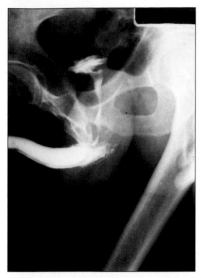

1106

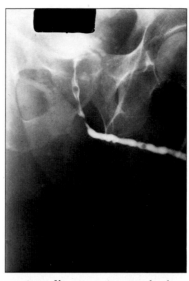

1107

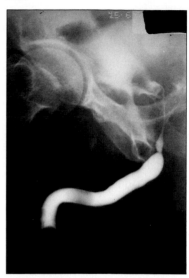

1105 Urethral stricture caused by inflammatory disease or trauma leads to symptoms of difficulty of micturition, straining to void, and a thin stream. Ascending urethrography will delineate the number, site, and length of the strictures. When very tight strictures are present or there is associated inflammation, extravasation may occur.

1106 Multiple anterior strictures.
1107 Tight stricture at the urethral bulb.

1108

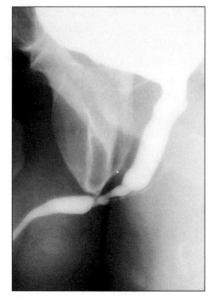

1109

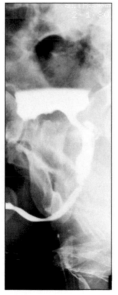

1110

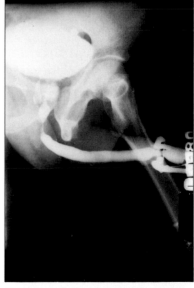

1108 Anterior urethral stricture in front of the bulb after gonococcal infection.

1109 Multiple strictures with associated diverticulum.

1110 Stricture at the level of the verumontanum with a false passage. These are usually iatrogenic after endoscopic manoeuvres.

1111

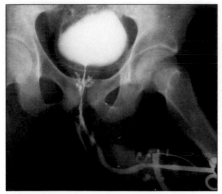

1111 Double stricture in the region of the urethral bulb. The prostatic ducts are filled with contrast.

1112

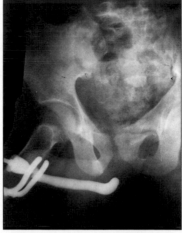

1112 Complete obstruction at the urethral bulb. Note the fractured pelvis.

1113

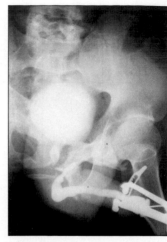

1113 Complete dissociation of urethra and bladder after extensive trauma.

1114

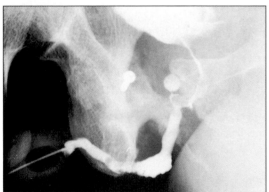

1114 Complex urethral stricture following major pelvic trauma.

1115

1115 Stricture with associated false passage after bouginage.

1116

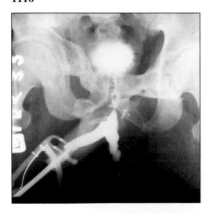

1116 Stricture with a fistula distal to a stricture.

1117

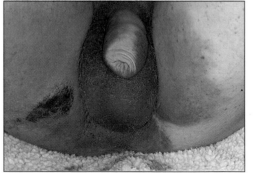

1117 Perineal trauma following astride injury in a window cleaner.

Perineal trauma is classically the result of falling astride. This leads to a gross perineal haematoma and can be followed by a bulbar stricture as occurred in this patient.

1118

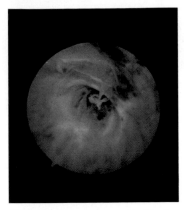

1118 Endoscopy reveals the inflamed urethral mucosal appearance at the face of the stricture. The mucosa is seen to be inflamed.

1119

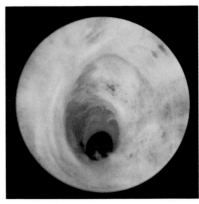

1119 Appearance of a scarred, fibrotic, and long-standing stricture.

1120

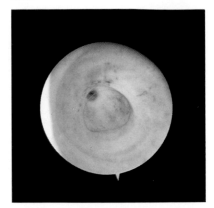

1120 A very tight stricture.

1121 A stricture with associated false passages.

1122 The healed chronic false passage in association with stricture.

1121

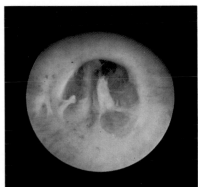

1122

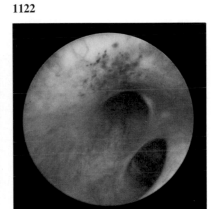

1123 Operative appearance of the gross scarring in urethral stricture.

1123

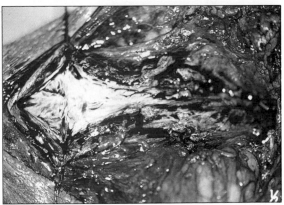

Urethral tumours

Urethral tumours are rare. Bleeding per urethram unassociated with micturition is the major presenting symptom. Viral lesions and occasionally papillary tumours are found in the anterior urethra and may protrude from within the external meatus.

Malignant urethral tumours—TNM clinical classification

T (primary tumour)

TX Primary tumour can not be assessed.
T0 No evidence of primary tumour.
Ta Noninvasive papillary, polypoid, or verrucous carcinoma.
Tis Carcinoma *in situ*.
T1 Tumour invades subepithelial connective tissue.

T2 Tumour invades corpus spongiosum or prostate or periurethral muscle.
T3 Tumour invades corpus cavernosum or beyond prostatic capsule or anterior vagina or bladder neck.
T4 Tumour invades other adjacent organs.

N

N0 No regional lymph node metastasis.
N1 Single < 2 cm.
N2 Single > 2–5 cm. Multiple < 5 cm.
N3 > 5 cm.

M

M0 No distant metastasis.
M1 Distant metastasis.

These tumours tend to arise in the posterior urethra, and present with bleeding per urethram rather than haematuria and symptoms of obstructed micturition.

1124

1125

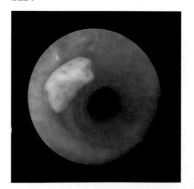

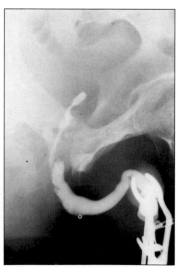

1124 Urethral tumour: benign endoscopy appearance.

1125, 1126, 1127 Ascending urethrography will reveal an irregular ragged stricture in the deep urethra indicating a malignant tumour. These lesions are highly malignant locally, but rarely metastasise and are therefore amenable to radical surgery.

1126

1127

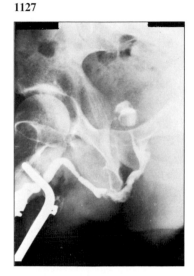

1128

1129

1128 Endoscopy reveals the irregular ragged appearance of a malignant tumour.

1129 The excised urethral tumour seen in 1128 is visible within the urethra.

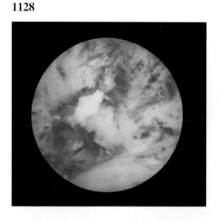

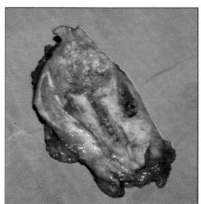

1130

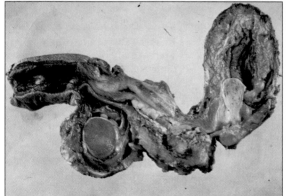

1131

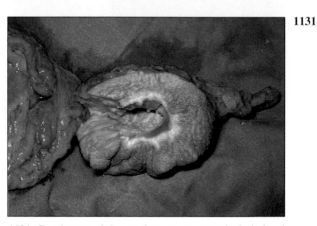

1130 Transitional carcinoma of the urethra. Tumour surrounds the bulbomembranous urethra over a 6 cm length. It is growing into the lumen of the urethra and is invading the root of the penis. Histology showed it to be a transitional carcinoma. There is also benign prostatic hypertrophy (median lobe) with evidence of bladder outflow obstruction.

1131 Carcinoma of the urethra occurs extensively in local tissues without distant metastases. Here the lesion is ulcerating through the perineal skin. This patient remained alive without recurrence 3 years after radical local surgery.

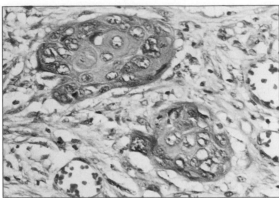

1132 Squamous cell carcinoma of the urethra. The section shows islands of large cells with eosinophilic cytoplasm and pleomorphic nuclei infiltrating through connective tissue. Although not making keratin, the cells resemble those of the Malpighian layer (prickle cell layer) of the skin. This is a poorly differentiated squamous cell carcinoma. *(H&E × 160)*

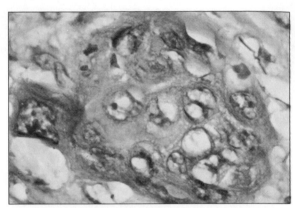

1133 Squamous cell carcinoma of urethra. Higher magnification of **1132** in which the desmosomes between some of the squamous cells are visible. *(H&E × 400)*

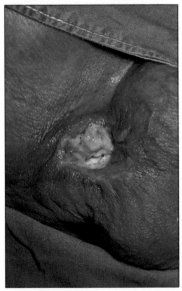

1134 The tumour grows extensively locally without metastasising distantly until very late in the disease process. However, fungation may occur through the perineal skin.

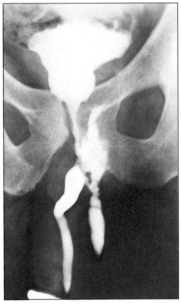

1135 Malignant fistula may occur in the urethra when malignant disease spreads locally from the rectum as shown in this ascending urethrogram.

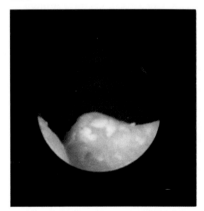

1136 Female urethral carcinoma is also rare. This endoscopic view shows an early lesion at the bladder neck. There was no tumour lesion in the bladder.

1137 Transitional cell carcinoma of the urethra exists in all the forms seen in the bladder. This tumour is part of a papillary transitional cell carcinoma. *(H&E × 160)*

1138 Caruncles are painful red swellings at the female external urethral meatus. They consist of inflamed vascular connective tissue covered with epithelium. Often one or other element predominates to give different histological pictures, but they are probably variants of the same process.

1137

1138

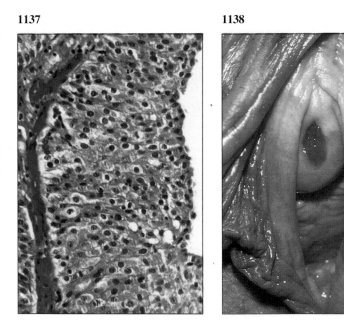

1139

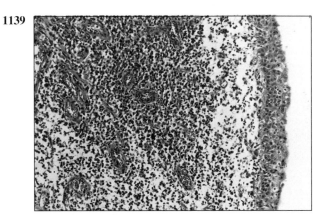

1139 A caruncle covered with transitional epithelium, but composed mainly of loose chronic inflammatory tissue with blood vessels and a heavy infiltrate of inflammatory cells. *(H&E × 64)*

1140

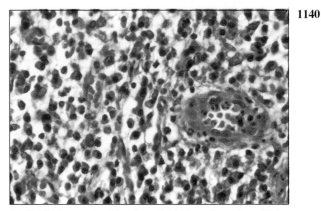

1140 Higher magnification of 1139 to show the cellular infiltrate composed mainly of plasma cells and one of the blood vessels with neutrophil polymorphonuclear leucocytes in its walls. *(H&E × 256)*

1141

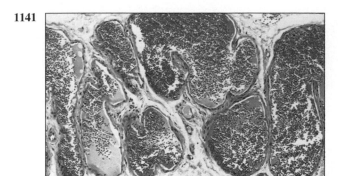

1142

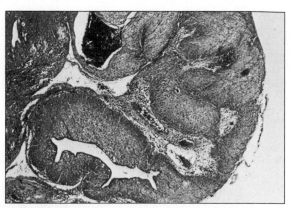

1141 Part of a caruncle composed largely of telangiectatic blood vessels and with little inflammatory cell reaction in the connective tissue. *(H&E × 64)*

1142 Part of a caruncle showing marked epithelial proliferation dipping down into the connective tissue. *(H&E × 64)*

11 Diseases of the penis and scrotum

Diseases of the penis may be classified as congenital, inflammatory, traumatic and neoplastic.

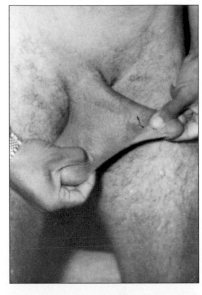

1143 The rare webbed penis.

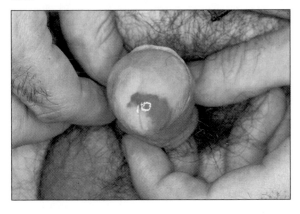

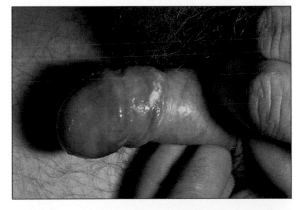

1144 and 1145 Balanitis. Inflammation of the glans penis usually occurs with an associated phimosis; the inflamed glans is viewed with the prepuce retracted. A more extensive lesion is shown in **1145**.

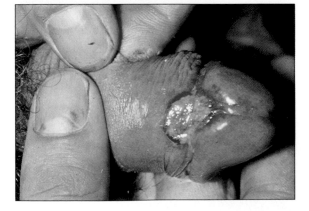

1146 The painless primary chancre of syphilis with its wash-leather base must be distinguished from a malignant ulcer.

1147

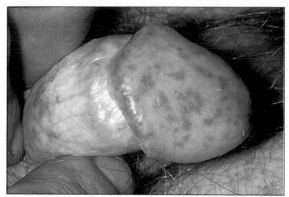

1147 Fungal infections may cause superficial penile lesions as in this patient with a monilial infection. The glans is a mottled purple colour.

1148

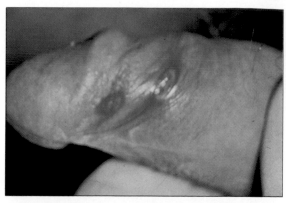

1148 Painful local ulcers with accompanying painful nodes occur in herpes. The early vascular lesion can be seen more proximal to the small ulcer.

1149

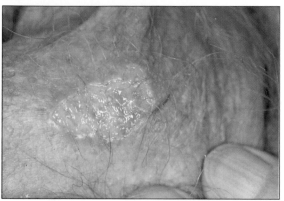

1149 A large erosive herpetic ulcer.

1150

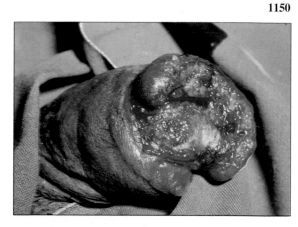

1150 Nonspecific chronic inflammation may produce massive penile necrosis.

1151

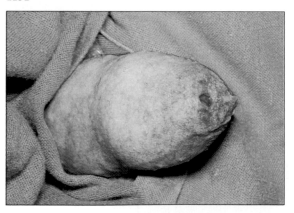

1151 Phimosis may be unaccompanied by infection but may cause mechanical pain with erection because of failure to retract the prepuce.

1152

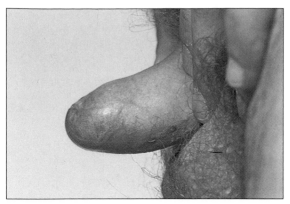

1153

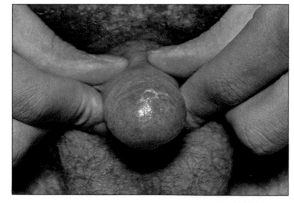

1152 and 1153 A severe degree of phimosis is shown in two views.

1154

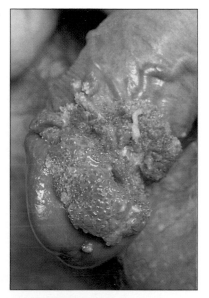

1154 Multiple papillary warts.

1155

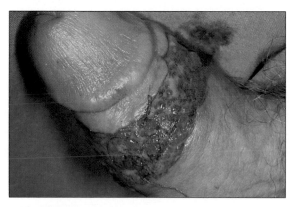

1155 Self-inflicted penile trauma.

Penile trauma can occur with degloving injuries due to accidents at work with machinery but may also be self-inflicted as in **1155** in which the patient attempted a home circumcision.

1156

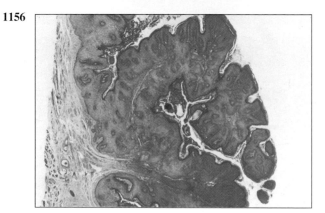

1156 Penile warts. Papillary outgrowths of hyperplastic stratified squamous epithelium. *(H&E × 64)*

1157

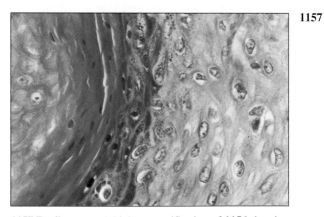

1157 Penile warts. A higher magnification of **1156** showing hyperkeratosis and parakeratosis (at the top of the field) overlying a prominent granular cell layer, with many cells containing keratohyaline granules and some cells being vacuolated. Beneath this zone is the acanthotic Malpighian (prickle cell) layer. *(H&E × 256)*

1158

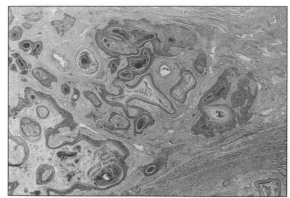

1158 Buschke-Löwenstein lesion. Occasionally large warty lesions are seen on the penis which grow into the underlying tissue and destroy it. The terms 'Buschke-Löwenstein lesions', 'giant condyloma accuminata', 'verrucous carcinoma' and 'carcinoma cuniculatum' are applied to such warty lesions which are well differentiated and which infiltrate but metastasise late or not at all. Some authors claim that these lesions can be distinguished as separate entities, while others group them together as squamous-cell neoplasms of low-grade malignancy. This section shows islands of well-differentiated squamous epithelium which are keratinising and extending into the erectile tissue of the penis. *(H&E × 64)*

1159

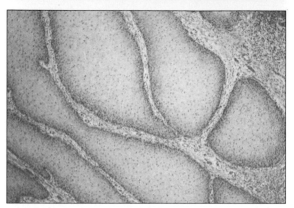

1159 Buschke-Löwenstein lesion. This section shows the pegs of well-differentiated squamous epithelium (this time nonkeratinising) dipping down into the connective tissue. It can be very difficult to distinguish a benign lesion from a malignant lesion of this type. *(H&E × 256)*

1161

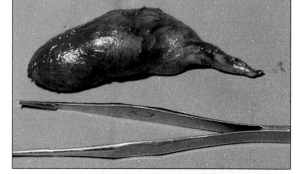

1162

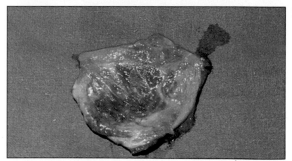

1160

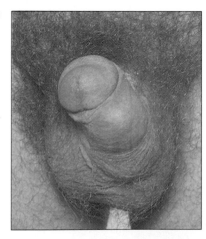

Rarely do benign swellings develop in the penis.

1160, 1161, 1162 and 1163 A dermoid cyst arising in the penile shaft.

1163

Ectopic testis

Occasionally the incompletely descended ectopic testis may lie beneath the skin of the penile shaft, producing the appearance of a tumour.

Gangrene of the penis

1164

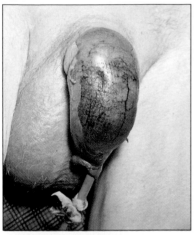

1164 Gangrene of the penis is very rare and almost always follows occlusive bands being placed around the penile shaft.

Penile trauma

1165

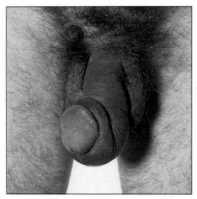

1165 Penile trauma, which is most frequently caused by coitus, will produce bruising and oedema with haematoma formation.

1166

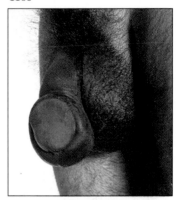

1166 If a corpus cavernosum is damaged, gross angulation may result.

1167

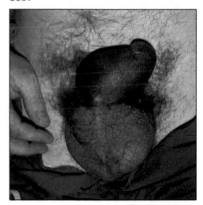

1167 Intense penile bruising may occur.

Priapism

1168

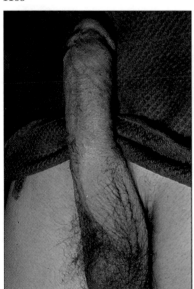

1169

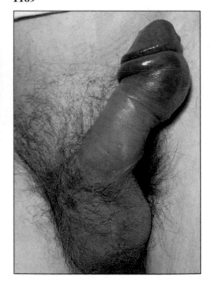

1168 and 1169 Priapism, in which the penile corpora only remain persistently turgid, is usually idiopathic but may accompany haematological disease such as sickle-cell disease and leukaemia. The glans is not involved in the condition. See p.258, **1170** for corpora cavernography.

1170

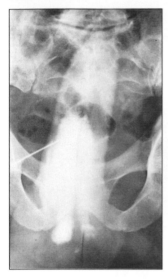

1170 Corpora cavernography in priapism shows failure of the dye to drain by the normal venous channels.

Investigation of impotence

1171   **1172**

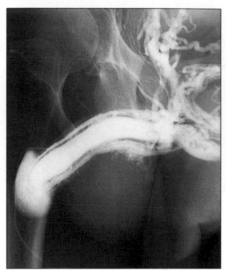

1171 Cavernogram in a patient with gross venous leak. There is also a leak into glans penis and corpus spongiosum.

1172 Anteroposterior view of region of the symphysis demonstrates gross venous leakage from the base of the corpora.

Cavernography is also very important in the investigation of impotence.

The two studies below can be compared with the normal papaverine-stimulated penile and colour Doppler flow.

1173

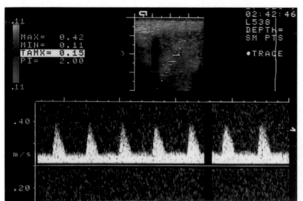

1174

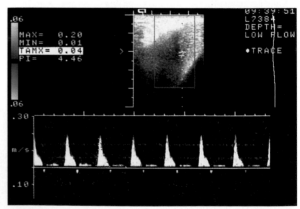

1173 Papaverine-stimulated colour Doppler study of the cavernosal arteries in a patient with a venous leak. Although maximum flow in systole is normal (0.42m/s), there is increased flow in diastole (0.11m/s).

1174 Papaverine-stimulated colour Doppler study of the cavernosal arteries in a patient with arterial insufficiency. There is poor maximum flow in systole (0.20m/s), but there is decreased flow in diastole (0.01m/s).

Peyronie's disease

1175 **Peyronie's disease** is distinguished by the presence of painful sometimes tender fibrous plaques arising in the walls of the corpora and leads to angulation of the penile shafts on erection. A plaque is demonstrated at surgery.

1175

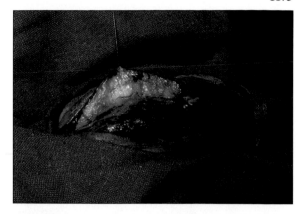

1176

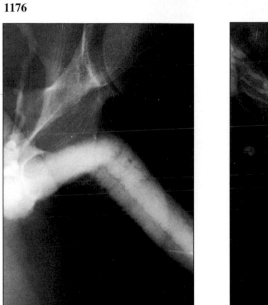

1177

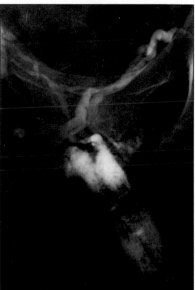

1176 Corpus cavernosogram demonstrates extreme angulation of shaft due to Peyronie plaque.

1177 Corpus cavernosogram demonstrating narrowing of corpora produced by this condition.

1178

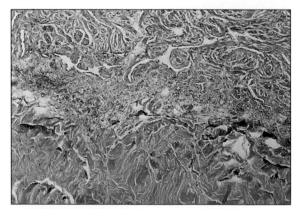

1179

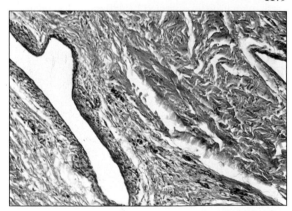

1178 Peyronie's disease. In this form of fibromatosis, proliferation of fibrous tissue (in the bottom area of the field) leads to obliteration of vessels and the development of a fibrous plaque in the corpora cavernosa. *(H&E × 26)*

1179 Peyronie's disease. The section shows the vascular channels of the corpora cavernosa being surrounded by dense fibrous tissue (stained green) and being obliterated. *(Masson's trichrome × 64)*

Paraphimosis

1180

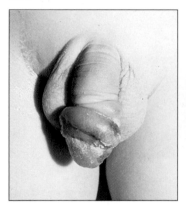

1181

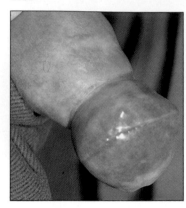

1180 Paraphimosis usually presents acutely when the retracted foreskin is not replaced and oedema is caused by the tight pre-coronal band.

1181 Paraphimosis. The condition is best seen in the lateral view. The tight band is clearly visible.

1182 and 1183 Paraphimosis. The condition may become chronic, causing severe local inflammation.

1184 Wart-like inflammatory changes occur when unsatisfactory long-term penile appliances are worn.

1182

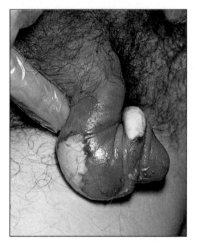

1183

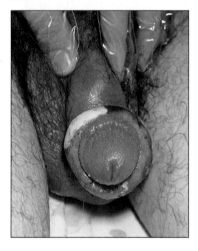

1184

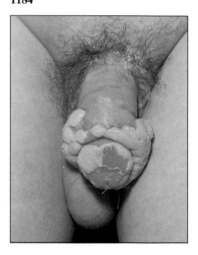

Balanitis xerotica obliterans is a dyskeratosis of the penis, which is manifested by inflammatory changes. In the very long term, these may become fibrotic and atrophic, leading to stenotic lesions of the distal urethra and occasionally progressing to carcinoma.

1185

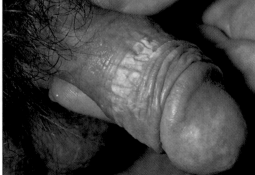

1185 The rugose, whitish appearance of the retracted prepuce.

1186

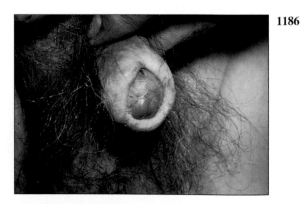

1186 The stenosing band at the edge of the foreskin.

1187

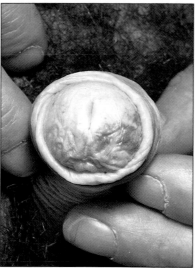

1188

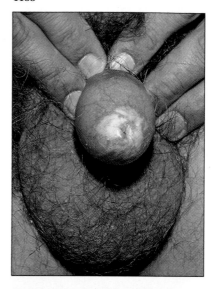

1187 Early telangiectasia of the glans with the rugose glandular appearance.

1188 Atrophic changes around the external meatus lead to stenosis.

1189

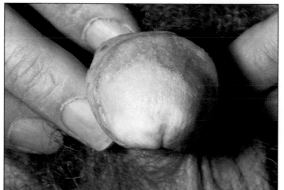

1189 Late atrophic changes in the glans.

1190

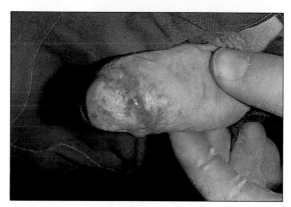

1190 Very late changes of gross telangiectasia and coronal obliteration.

1191

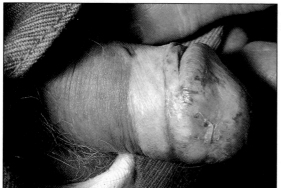

1191 Similar changes with a white preputial band.

1192

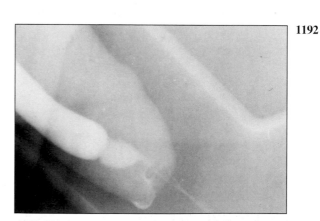

1192 Urethrogram showing distal urethral and meatal stenosis.

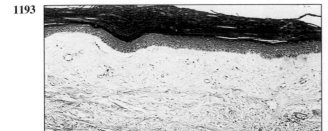

1193

1193 Balanitis xerotica obliterans. Histologically this condition is the same as lichen sclerosus et atrophicus. There is hyperkeratosis, atrophy of the Malpighian (prickle cell) layer of the epithelium, loss of the rete ridges and presence of a hyalinised band of collagen beneath the epithelium. *(H&E × 64)*

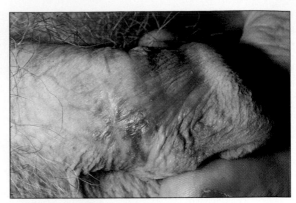

1194

1194 Carcinoma *in situ* lesions include Paget's disease of the penis and the erythroplasia of Queyrat. The indolent slightly raised erythematous patches of Paget's disease can be seen.

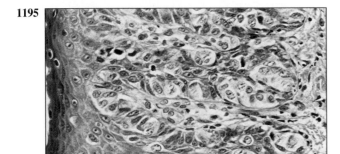

1195

1195 Paget's disease occurs rarely on the penis giving a histological appearance similar to that in the nipple. In the epithelium there is widespread infiltration of the basal layer and adjacent layers of the epithelium with large cells with pale cytoplasm – Paget's cells. *(H&E × 160)*

1196

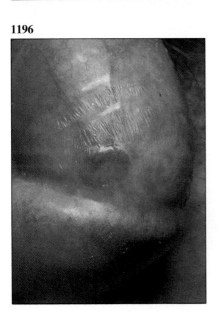

1197

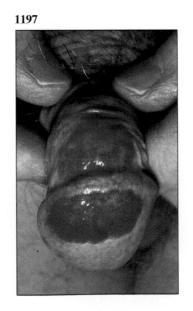

1196 Queyrat's erythroplasia. Persistent areas of reddened skin which are resistant to local treatment raise the possibility of such diagnoses, which can only be proved by biopsy. *(H&E original mag. × 80)*

1197 Very extensive Queyrat's erythroplasia.

1198

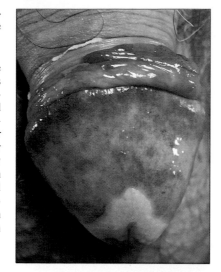

1199

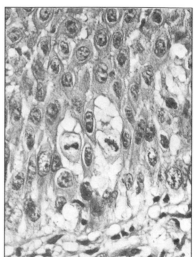

1198 Extreme Queyrat's erythroplasia. Note the sclerosis around the meatus.

1199 Queyrat's erythroplasia. The histological appearance of Queyrat's erythroplasia is that of a thickened dysplastic epithelium with cellular atypia and prominent mitoses. Infiltrating squamous-cell carcinoma develops in about 10 per cent of cases. The appearances are similar to Bowen's disease. Histologically it may not be possible to distinguish them with certainty. Bowen's disease is associated with other malignancies, whereas Queyrat's is not. Bowen's disease may occur on the shaft whereas Queyrat's is usually on the glans and prepuce. *(H&E × 256)*

1200

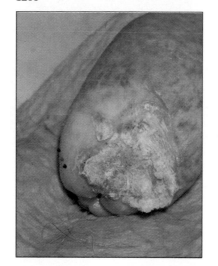

1201

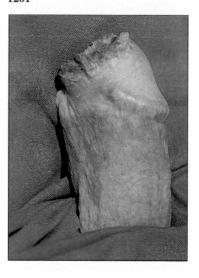

1200 Horns of keratin may arise on the glans penis. This condition of hyperkeratosis is premalignant.

1201 The glans may sometimes produce bizarre forms of tissue.

1202

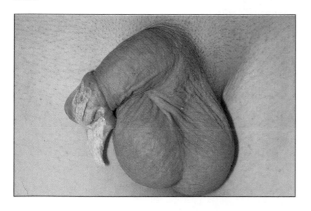

1203

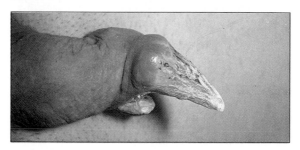

1202 and 1203 Examples of penile horn.

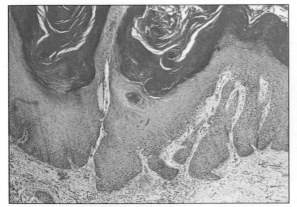

1204 Penile horn. The section shows hyperkeratosis, para-keratosis and acanthosis. There is little atypicality of the epithelial cells. *(H&E × 64)*

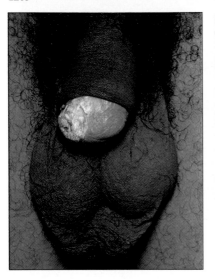
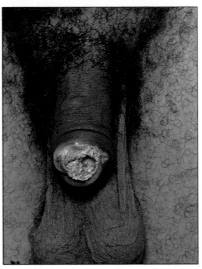

1205 and 1206 Penile horn progressing to a frank carcinoma in the same patient over a 2-year period.

Tumours of the penis and prepuce

TNM clinical classification

T (primary tumour)

TX	Primary tumour cannot be assessed
TO	No evidence of primary tumour
Tis	Carcinoma *in situ*
Ta	Noninvasive verrucous carcinoma
T1	Tumour invades subepithelial connective tissue
T2	Tumour invades corpus spongiosum or cavernosum
T3	Tumour invades urethra or prostate
T4	Tumour invades other adjacent structures

N (regional lymph nodes)

NX	Regional lymph nodes cannot be assessed
NO	No regional lymph node metastasis
N1	Metastasis in a single superficial inguinal lymph node
N2	Metastasis in multiple or bilateral superficial inguinal lymph nodes
N3	Metastasis in deep inguinal or pelvic lymph node(s), unilateral or bilateral

M (distant metastasis)

MO	No distant metastases
M1	Distant metastases

1207 Carcinomas may arise from the undersurface of the prepuce and present growing from beneath it.

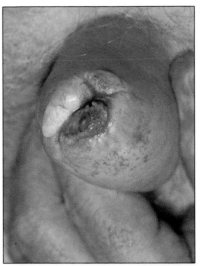

1207

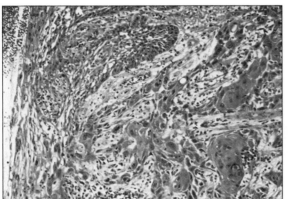

1208

1208 Prepuce: squamous carcinoma. The irregular squamous epithelium of the surface is on the left. Disordered strands of epithelium are invading down into the connective tissue. *(H&E × 64)*

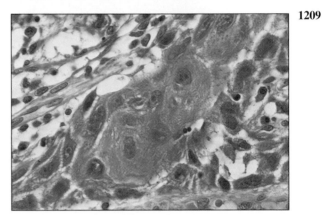

1209

1209 Prepuce: squamous carcinoma. A higher magnification of part of **1208,** showing an irregular island of squamous epithelium in connective tissue, with a few associated chronic inflammatory cells. *(H&E × 256)*

1210 Penile carcinoma. When a purulent or sanguino-purulent discharge occurs from beneath the phimosed prepuce of the adult, then circumcision may be necessary to reveal the underlying penile carcinoma.

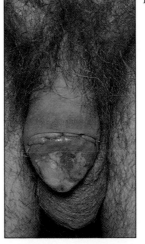

1210

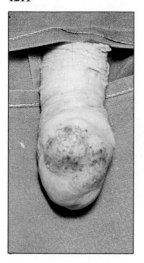

Stages of penile carcinomas

1211 An early lesion.

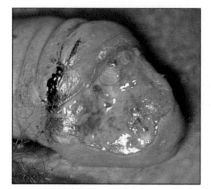

1212 Local destruction of glans.

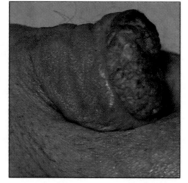

1213 Bulky lesion involving the shaft.

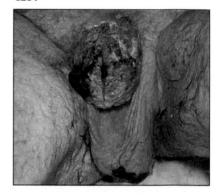

1214 Erosion of the corpora may lead to torrential haemorrhages as in this patient.

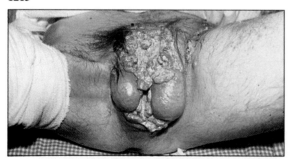

1215 Gross destruction of the whole penile shaft and involving the scrotum.

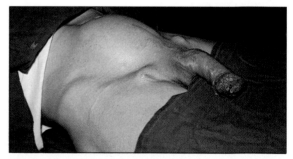

1216 Penile carcinoma. In the elderly, slow progression, fear and neglect, may lead to patients failing to present with penile carcinomas until they go into acute urinary retention as can be seen here. Groin gland metastases are well shown here.

1217 Scrotal wart.

1218 Histology of a wart. Papillary outgrowths of acanthotic stratified squamous epithelium showing no evidence of malignancy.

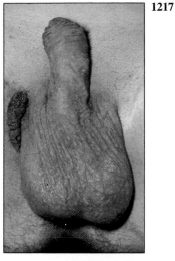

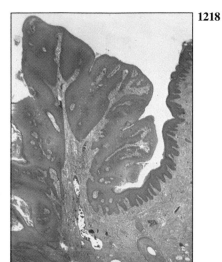

1219 Epithelial cysts of scrotal skin are common and a small typical cyst is shown.

1220 Section of a small cyst filled with keratin. Sometimes the cysts rupture and stimulate a foreign body giant-cell reaction in the surrounding tissue. Sometimes only cyst contents remain, with little or no reaction. *(H&E × 16)*

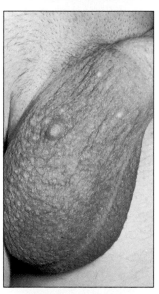

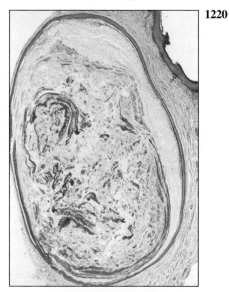

1221 and 1222 Oil cancers of the scrotum are now a rare form of occupational cancer, sometimes presenting in workers in the engineering and textile industries. An early and late form are shown. The histological pattern is no different to any squamous-cell skin carcinoma despite the chemical aetiology.

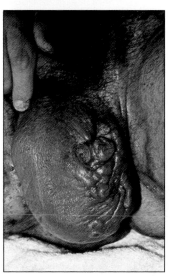

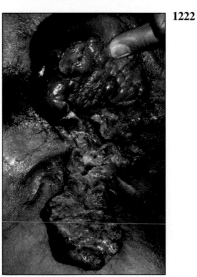

1223

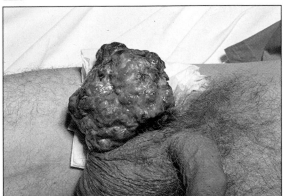

1224

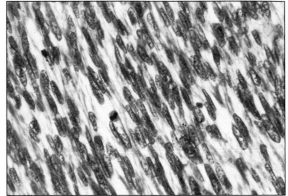

1223 Other scrotal tumours are rare and a spindle-cell sarcoma is shown.

1224 Scrotum: spindle-cell sarcoma. Sections show that the tumour is made up of sheets of poorly differentiated cells which are elongated. Mitoses are prominent. *(H&E × 256)*

12 Diseases of the testis

Enlargement of the scrotal contents is of great clinical importance because of the difficulties with differential diagnosis and the necessity for early confirmation of testicular tumour. Simple painless enlargements are usually found to be cystic. Hydroceles are normally primary (idiopathic), transluminated brilliantly and unless very lax the testis cannot be palpated. Secondary hydroceles are associated with testicular pathology.

Ultrasonography has now become an integral part of the investigation and management of scrotal lesions.

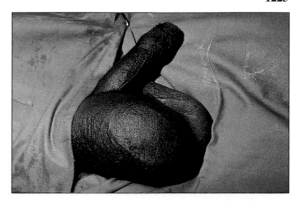

1225 A hydrocele enlarges the scrotum and, unlike an inguinal hernia, the upper extent of the swelling can be easily determined.

1226

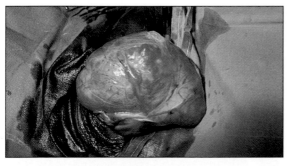

1226 When the scrotal skin is reflected the hydrocele and its coverings are displayed.

1227

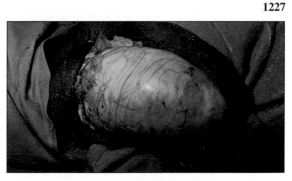

1227 Further dissection displays the thin wall of the hydrocele sac.

1228

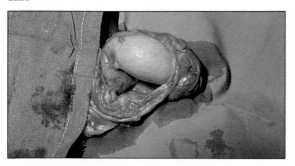

1228 When the sac is opened the normal testis is visible.

1229

1229 In very long-standing hydroceles a rare complication of calcification of the wall may occur. Usually this is post-traumatic.

Appendix testis

1230

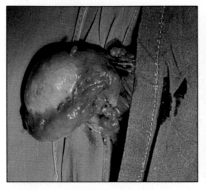

1230 A testicular appendage, the hydatid of Morgagni, can be seen at the upper pole. These appendages can undergo torsion.

1231

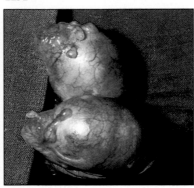

1231 These appendages may be bilateral.

1232

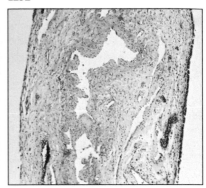

1232 This vestigial structure (also called the hydatid of Morgagni) is derived from the upper end of the paramesonephric duct. It is composed of a core of vascular connective tissue and is normally covered by columnar or cuboidal epithelium. *(H&E × 26)*

1233

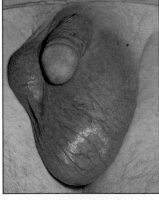

1233 The cyst of epididymis will usually have a similar scrotal contour of the hydrocele, but occasionally the testis may be observed below the cyst.

1234

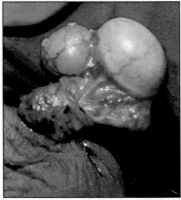

1234 Careful palpation will show that the testis can be palpated separately from the small cyst, here shown at exploration.

1235

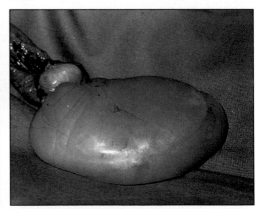

1235 A large epididymal cyst. Some contain spermatozoa and therefore can be termed spermatoceles. These tend to transilluminate less brilliantly than epididymal cysts and primary hydroceles.

1236

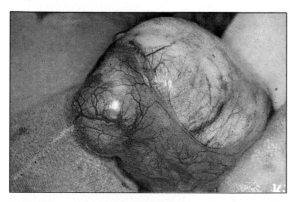

1237

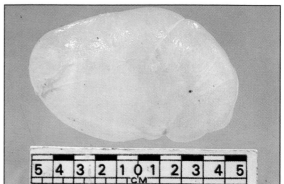

1236 This small epididymal cyst has arisen close to the body of the testis in the globus major.

1237 Excised cyst of epididymis.

1238

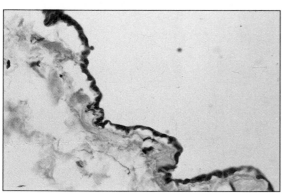

1239

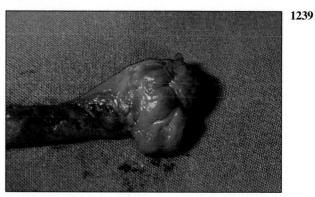

1238 Spermatoceles. These cysts contain sperm in the fluid but these are not seen in histological preparations. The epithelial lining is similar to a hydrocele and is usually cuboidal, but this may be attenuated to form a flattened lining: occasionally a pseudostratified appearance is seen. There is loose connective tissue outside. *(H&E × 160)*

1239 Solid benign lesions may arise in the epididymis as painless swellings and cause difficulty with diagnosis.

1240

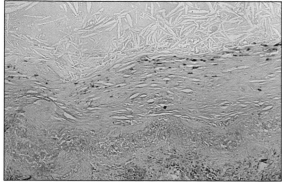

1241

> **Hydrocele fluid content**
>
> Clear
> Specific gravity of more than 1020
> Inorganic salts
> Albumin
> Fibrinogen
> Cholesterol

1242

> **Epididymal cyst fluid content**
>
> Opalescent
> Low specific gravity less than 1005
> A small amount of protein or no protein
> Cells and occasional spermatozoa

1240 Histology reveals a fibrous nodule which may have followed rupture of a cyst.

1241 and 1242 The fluid aspirated from the cystic lesions of the scrotum differs according to the type of lesion.

1243

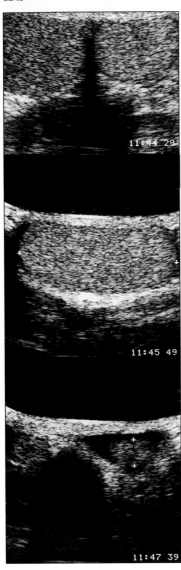

1243 Normal ultrasound studies of the testes shown transversely and longitudinally, together with the normal epididymis for comparison.

1244

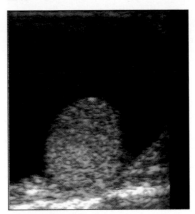

1244 Ultrasound of primary hydrocele with normal testes surrounded by fluid.

1245

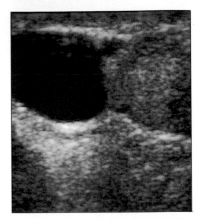

1245 Ultrasound of benign epididymal cyst adjacent and attached to body of the testis.

1246

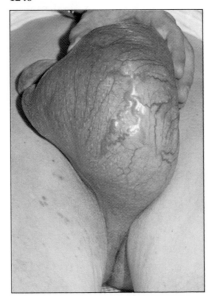

1246 Paratesticular lipoma. This massive tumour, which felt lobulated, rubbery and did not transilluminate, presented in the scrotum and caused congestion of the scrotal veins.

1247

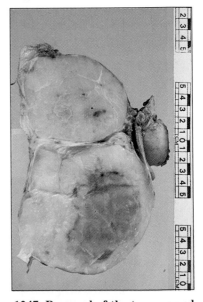

1247 Removal of the tumour and testis, to which it was closely adherent, revealed a large, lobulated, yellowish mass. Histology revealed mature adipose tissue with areas of fat necrosis. Despite the size of the mass, there was no evidence of malignancy.

Epididymitis

1248

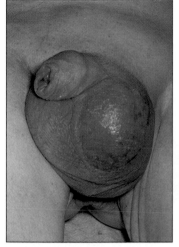

1249

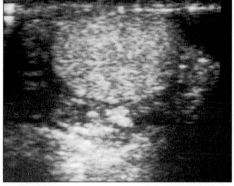

1249 Ultrasound. Longitudinal sections showing normal testis with very swollen epididymis.

1250

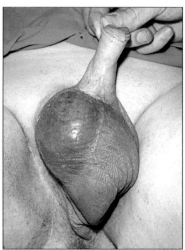

1248 Epididymitis. The enlarged inflamed epididymis and body of testis with associated scrotal erythema. A complication of urinary tract infection which can pose diagnostic problems since torsion may produce a similar clinical picture.

1250 Torsion. This lesion, which can rarely be bilateral, leads to a true urological emergency and may be very difficult to diagnose. In the infant, torsion of the whole cord may result in testicular infarction. In the adolescent, torsion of the body of the testis or of the body and epididymis occurs within the tunica vaginalis. In this condition the testis may lie horizontally, the so-called 'bell-clapper' testis. Diagnosis can be very difficult as the onset may not be dramatic and the pain initially not severe. When lying high in the scrotum the diagnosis may be easier to reach but this condition is very readily confused with epididymo-orchitis. If torsion is suspected, exploration is imperative as there are only 6–8 hours from onset to irreversible infarction in most cases.

Torsion

1251

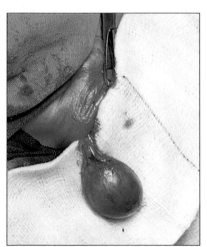

1251 The torted testis delivered at operation.

1252 Torsion: the whole cord is twisted here (formalin fixed).

1252

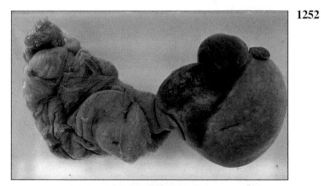

1253 The resected specimen is seen to be infarcted (formalin fixed).

1253

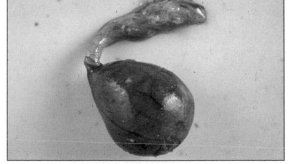

1254

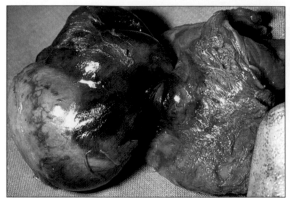

1254 The body of the testis is twisted within the tunica vaginalis and is deeply congested.

1255

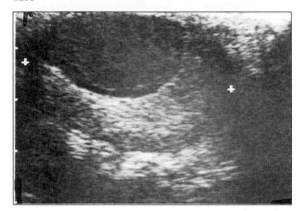

1256

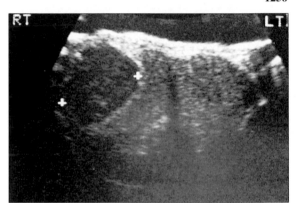

1255 and 1256 Ultrasound. Longitudinal (**1255**) and transverse (**1256**) studies of testis showing swollen epididymis and lower echogenicity of testis indicating inflammation as a result of torsion. The absence of blood flow can be confirmed by Doppler studies.

1257

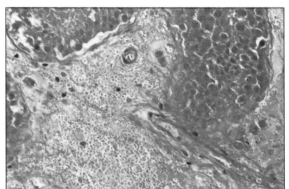

1257 This section shows the infarction which follows torsion. The ghost outlines of dead tubules are seen in the upper part of the field; haemorrhage is present in the oedematous loose connective tissue between. *(H&E × 50)*

1258

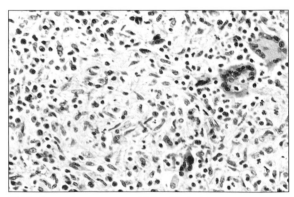

1258 Granulomatous orchitis. Clinically presenting as a solid enlarged body of testis, this inflammatory lesion may be mistaken for a tumour both clinically and histologically. It is characterised by a chronic inflammatory-cell infiltration in which there are aggregates of histiocytes, some of which may be multinucleate. These granulomas are noncaseating and are thought to be a reaction to the contents of ruptured tubules. It is important to exclude tuberculosis. *(H&E × 160)*

Varicocoele

1259

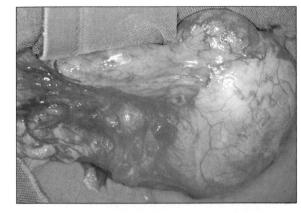

1259 Varicocele. Classically the patient describes the feeling of a 'bag of worms' within his scrotum. These varicose veins transmit a cough impulse and arise from the pampiniform plexus, with or without a cremasteric element.

1260 The vascular anatomy of the cord.

1261 Stage I varicocele. The cremasteric veins are not involved.

1262 Stage II varicocele. The cremasteric veins are involved.

1260

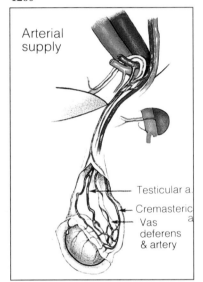

1261

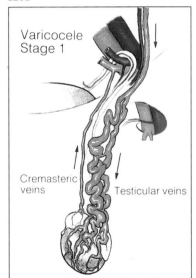

1262

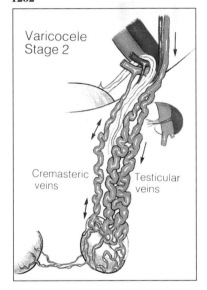

1263

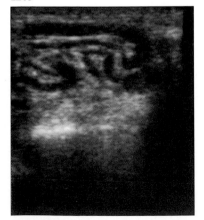

1264

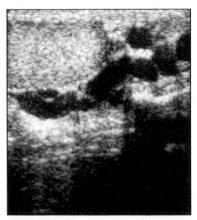

1265

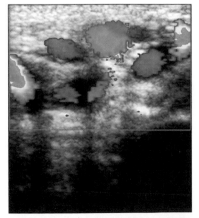

1263 Ultrasound of varicocele.

1264 High resolution ultrasound of a patient with a varicocele. There are perpiginous structures surrounding the lower pole.

1265 Effect of increasing venous pressure. When the patient is asked to perform the Valsalva manoeuvre, increased blood flow is seen within these structures on colour Doppler, indicating that this is a significant varicocele.

1266

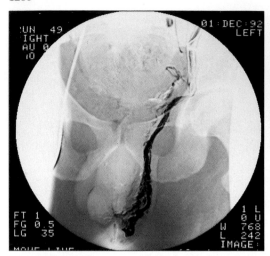

1267

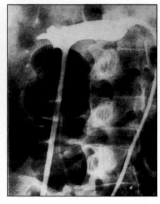

1268

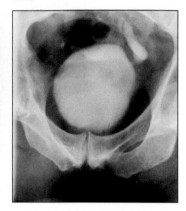

1267 Selective renal venography showing incompetence of the testicular vein valves.

1268 An enormous varicocele pushing up the ureter to the fundus of the bladder.

1266 Digital subtraction venogram of the left testicular vein showing the large varicocele.

1269

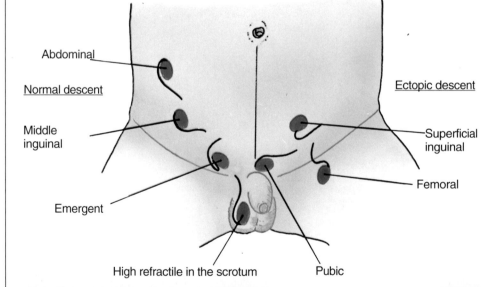

Abdominal

Normal descent

Middle inguinal

Emergent

High refractile in the scrotum

Pubic

Ectopic descent

Superficial inguinal

Femoral

1269 Testicular maldescent. Diagram showing sites of incomplete and ectopic descent. Rarely, penile and perineal ectopic testes are also found.

1270

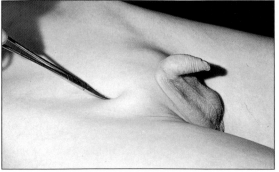

1270 The incompletely descended testis can be seen in the groin with the empty scrotum below.

1271

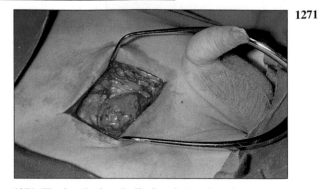

1271 The inguinal testis displayed at exploration.

1272

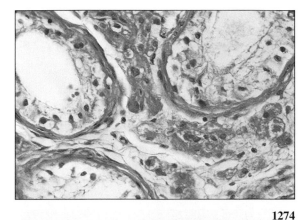

1272 The tubules in this specimen are lined by Sertoli cells and no spermatogenesis is apparent. The tubular basement membranes are hyalinised and there is peritubular fibrosis. Interstitial cells are prominent. *(H&E × 160)*

1273

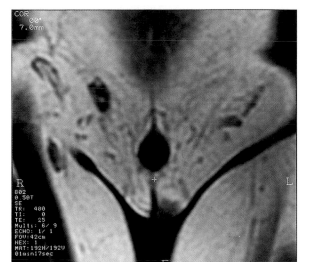

1274

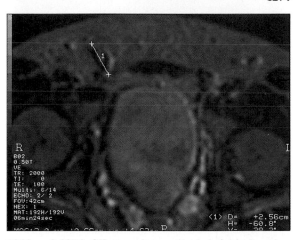

1273 and 1274 CT scanning maybe helpful in locating impalpable testes. The axial and coronal CT scan locate this impalpable right testis within the inguinal canal. The size of the testis can also be accurately assessed.

Testicular tumours

These tumours most commonly occur in men in their twenties and thirties. Although classically the tumour presents as an enlarging painless but heavy feeling testis, confusion often occurs in diagnosis because it has not been widely appreciated that more than one-third of the patients present with pain in the testis. Other presentations include the metastatic spread to the lungs and para-aortic nodes found at routine chest X-ray or on abdominal examination. It can also be an incidental finding during the investigation of infertility, either clinically or as an unsuspected lesion at testicular biopsy.

1275

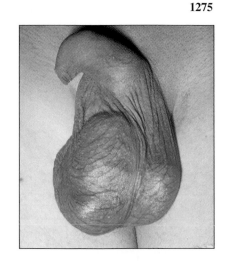

1275 At inspection the right testis is seen to be enlarged. The normal epididymis can normally be palpated. It is essential to differentiate between tumours and epididymo-orchitis, because both may present with pain. If a secondary hydrocele is present, it is usually small.

Investigation is determined by the mode of spread by the lymphatics to the para-aortic nodes and the bloodstream to the lungs and other organs.

Investigations: testicular tumours

1 Ultrasound.
2 Chest X-ray with whole lung tomography if CT scanning not available.
3 Lymphangiography.
4 IVU.
5 CT scanning.
6 Ultrasound of liver.
7 Blood markers: a) Serum alpha fetoprotein (AFP) – normal range: 1–10μg/1. b) Beta human chorionic gonadotrophin (ßHCG) – normal range: 1–2 μg/1.

8 Serum placental alkaline phosphatase (PlAB). Normal values < 0.5 units/l in non-smokers; < 1.5 units/l in smokers. This isoenzyme may also be used as an immunohistochemical marker in tissue sections of germ cell tumours
9 Liver function tests.
10 Renal function tests.
11 Full blood count.

1276

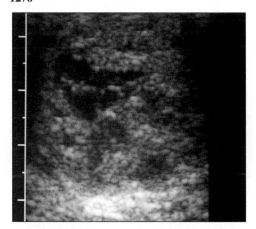

1276 Ultrasound of testicular tumour. Ultrasound of large testis shows a heterogeneous echo pattern typical of a testicular tumour and particularly found in teratomas as this proved to be.

The specimens for the estimation of the markers must be taken before orchiectomy. Although the AFP is seldom raised in pure seminomas its elevation when a seminoma has been found in the resected specimen suggests that there is in fact a mixed tumour or the occasional situation of liver metastases from a pure seminoma. The AFP principally rises in the yolk-sac tumour, and ßHCG in the chorion carcinoma. These markers will fall when all tumour is eradicated and are thus very valuable in demonstrating the presence of occult metastases which cannot be shown by other techniques. The importance of the normal plasma half-life of AFP at 5 days and ßHCG at 24–36 hours must be emphasised as the most significant method of assessing active disease, rather than their absolute values.

1277

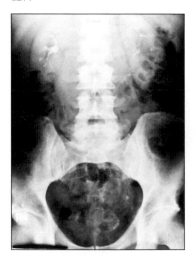

1278

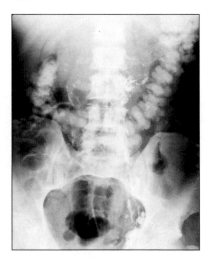

1279

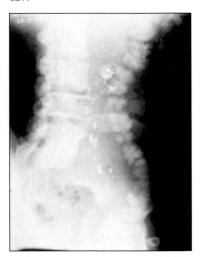

1277 IVU. The kidneys may be displaced laterally and rotated outwards by a para-aortic mass of glands.

1278 and 1279 Lymphangiography will confirm enlarged and abnormal lymph nodes with metastases. The dye in the colon is from the IVU carried out before the lymphogram. A lateral view is also shown.

1280

1280 IVU of a patient with para-aortic lymphadenopathy secondary to testicular teratoma obstructing the left kidney.

Assessment of para-aortic nodes is now best carried out by CT scanning which has replaced ultrasound in the accurate assessment of para-aortic nodes.

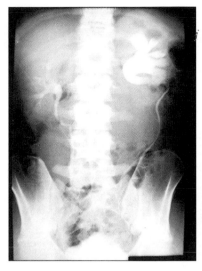

1281

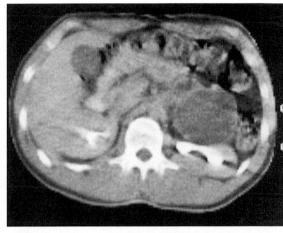

1281 CT scan of the patient in 1280, demonstrating para-aortic node mass and hydronephrotic left kidney.

1282

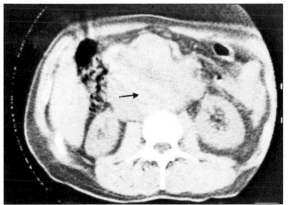

1282 CT scans confirm the presence of a vast mass of metastatic para-aortic nodes (arrowed).

1283

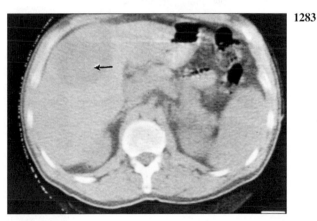

1283 The liver may be involved and the CT scan here shows liver metastases from a seminoma (arrowed).

1284

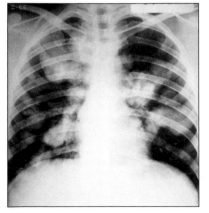

1284 Pulmonary metastases may be the presenting sign of testicular tumours.

1285

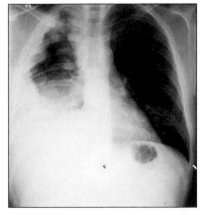

1285 Gross metastatic pulmonary disease may result from progression of the condition with pleural involvement.

1286

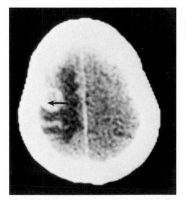

1286 Cerebral metastases may also be found and confirmed here by CT scan. Unilateral neurological symptoms and signs should alert the clinician to this possibility (arrowed).

1287

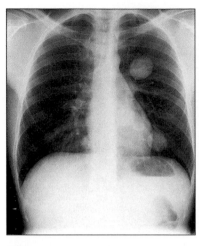

1287 Chest X-ray of patient who presented with a testicular teratoma in 1980. The lung metastases have remained static since treatment with chemotherapy, and are clearly mature teratoma.

1288

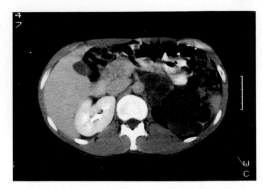

1288 CT scan showing left hydronephrosis and large gland mass in para-aortic region obstructing left kidney.

1289

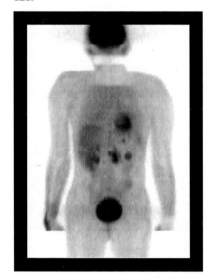

1290

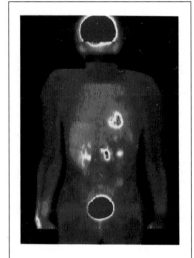

Positron emission tomography (PET) is valuable in localising soft tissue metastatic disease and can demonstrate inactive metastases.

1289 and 1290 PET scans showing active para-aortic node mass on left; two negative shadows in left lung field confirm these to be mature teratoma deposits.

1291

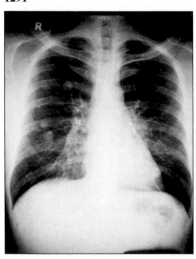

1292

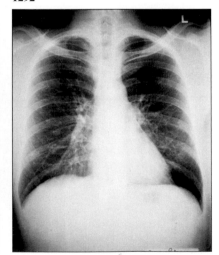

1291 Spontaneous regression of pulmonary metastases in testicular tumour is rare but recognised, following removal of the primary tumour. Multiple secondaries are seen in the lung fields.

1292 In this patient further pulmonary metastases developed subsequently. But here the lung fields have cleared following orchiectomy alone.

1293

1294

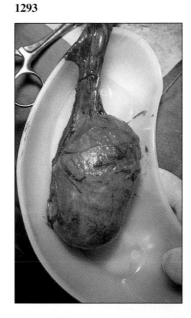

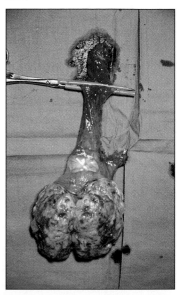

1293 The diagnosis is only proved by exploration. The groin is explored and the cord occluded with a noncrushing clamp. This expanded testis with its engorged veins is obviously grossly pathological.

1294 The excised testis is bisected and the tumour displayed.

1295

Testicular tumours can be present at birth and may occur in early life.

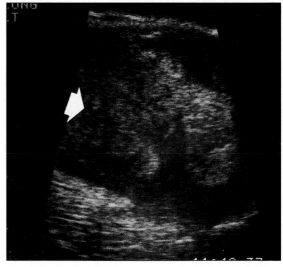

1295 Testicular ultrasound of 1-year-old child demonstrating tumour.

1296 Macroscopic specimen of tumour from the patient in 1295.

1297 Section through the testicular cell tumour shown in 1296 The section shows solid spindle cell areas with cavities lined by attentuated epithelium similar to the rare granulosa cell tumour. (*H&E × 80*)

1296

1297

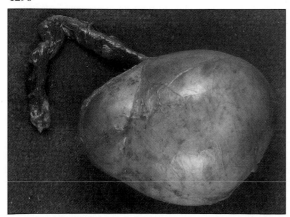

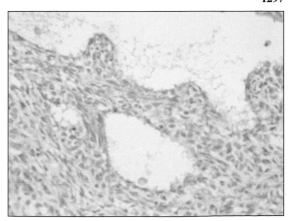

TNM pathological classification

T (primary tumour)

TX Primary tumour cannot be assessed (if no radical orchidectomy has been performed, TX is used).

TO No evidence of primary tumour (e.g. histological scar in testis).

Tis Intratubular tumour: preinvasive cancer.

T1 Tumour limited to testis, including rete testis.

T2 Tumour invades beyond tunica albuginea or into epididymis.

T3 Tumour invades spermatic cord.

T4 Tumour invades scrotum.

N (regional lymph nodes)

N1 Single node <2cm.

N2 Single node >2cm to 5cm. Multiple <5cm.

N3 >5cm.

M (distant metastasis)

MO No distant metastases.

M1 Distant metastases.

1298

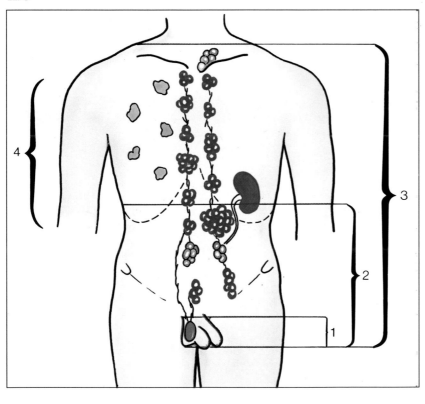

1298 Clinical staging of testicular tumours.

Stage 1 The tumour is confined to the testis.

Stage 2 There is involvement of the abdominal lymph nodes which are either manually palpable or demonstrated by radiological or other invest-igations.

Stage 3 Involved nodes above and below the diaphragm.

Stage 4 Extranodal metastases.

Primary tumours of the testis

Classification of testicular tumours is difficult because the conventional basis of histological typing, namely the cell of origin of the tumour, is hard to define when dealing with tumours which differentiate along many different lines. The main problem occurs with the definition of 'teratoma' and which tumours to include in this group:

Seminoma	Typical (well or poorly differentiated) Spermatocytic
Teratoma	Differentiated Intermediate Undifferentiated Trophoblastic
Combined seminoma and teratoma	
Yolk-sac tumour	
Others:	including interstitial cell tumour, Sertoli-cell tumour, gonadoblastoma, lymphoma, connective-tissue tumours.

Nomenclature of germ-cell tumours

The nomenclature of tumours which are believed to arise from testicular germ cells is not universally agreed. Most classifications distinguish seminoma and its subtypes from the others. Significant differences occur in the labelling of the nonseminoma group.

British classifications group the nonseminomas together as teratomas and distinguish them on the basis of:
● Embryonic or extra-embryonic differentiation (the latter includes trophoblastic and yolk-sac elements);
● The degree of differentiation of the embryonic elements.
American nomenclature reserves the term 'teratoma' for those tumours containing recognisable tissue of more than one germ layer. Less well-differentiated tumours which nevertheless have a poorly differentiated epithelial or embryonic appearance are called 'embryonal carcinoma'. Tumours with trophoblastic differentiation are named 'choriocarcinoma', whether or not other elements are present (see Table 8).

The so-called orchioblastoma (or adenocarcinoma of the infant testis) is now recognised as yolk-sac differentiation of a germ-cell tumour. This pattern of differentiation is more and more frequently recognised in adult germ-cell tumours.

* **Table 8.** Equivalent terms in different teratoma classifications.

Testicular tumour panel 1975	Armed Forces Institute of Pathology Fascicle 1973 (Mostofi & Price)	WHO 1975
Teratoma differentiated	Teratoma mature immature	Teratoma mature immature
Malignant teratoma intermediate	Embryonal carcinoma with teratoma, with or without other elements	Teratoma with malignant transformation Embryonal carcinoma and teratoma
Malignant teratoma undifferentiated	Embryonal carcinoma Adult Infantile Polyembryoma	Embryonal carcinoma
Malignant teratoma trophoblastic	Choriocarcinoma with or without embryonal carcinoma	Choriocarcinoma with or without embryonal carcinoma or other germ-cell tumour

*Pathology of the Testis, (Ed.) R.C.B. Pugh, Blackwell, 1976.

1299

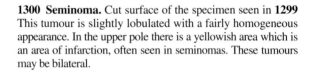

1299 Seminoma. Orchidectomy specimen. An enlarged testis but with no evidence of invasion through the tunica vaginalis.

1300

1300 Seminoma. Cut surface of the specimen seen in **1299** This tumour is slightly lobulated with a fairly homogeneous appearance. In the upper pole there is a yellowish area which is an area of infarction, often seen in seminomas. These tumours may be bilateral.

1301

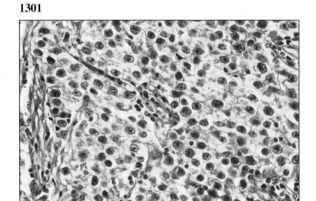

1301 Seminoma: well differentiated (typical). The tumour is composed of sheets of cells with delicate cytoplasm with large round nuclei and prominent nucleoli. There are scattered lymphocytes in the background and fine connective tissue bands often run between the tumour cells. *(H&E × 160)*

1302

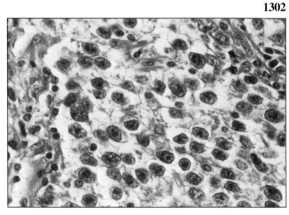

1302 Seminoma: well differentiated (typical). Higher magnification of the tumour seen in **1301**. The tumour cells are fairly regular and mitoses are infrequent (none in this field). Though the cytoplasm is delicate the cell boundaries are well seen. *(H&E × 256)*

1303

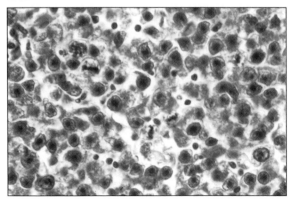

1303 Seminoma: (poorly differentiated). This tumour is similar to the typical seminoma on naked-eye examination, but microscopically it is different. Most important is the prominence of mitoses (five are present in this field), and there is also greater irregularity in the nuclei. The prognosis of these tumours is worse than for well-differentiated seminomas. These are sometimes called anaplastic seminomas. *(H&E × 256)*

1304

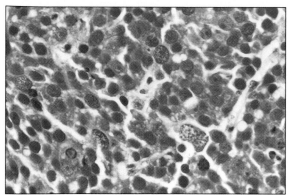

1304 Seminoma: spermatocytic. This tumour is distinguished from typical seminoma because of its histological appearances and better prognosis. Most of the cells are regular and have a round nucleus and eosinophilic cytoplasm. Other cells resemble secondary spermatocytes. A third type is a very large cell. *(H&E × 256)*

1305

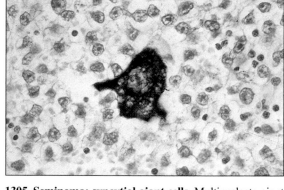

1305 Seminoma: syncytial giant cells. Multinucleate giant cells, resembling syncytial trophoblast are occasionally seen in seminomas. By immunohistology they can be shown to contain human chorionic gonadotrophin (HCG). At the moment their significance is not known. *(Immunoperoxidase for β subunit of HCG. × 160)*

1306

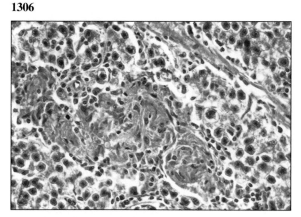

1306 Seminoma: granulomatous reaction. This section shows a seminoma, but in the centre of the field is a collection of large cells with plentiful eosinophilic cytoplasm, some of which are multinucleate. This is a giant-cell granuloma, a similar lesion to that seen in inflammatory conditions such as sarcoidosis. Lymphocytic infiltration and granulomata are thought to be host responses to the presence of the tumour. *(H&E × 160)*

1307

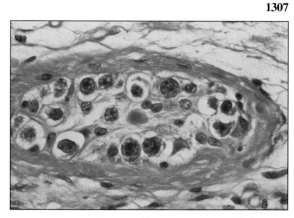

1307 Seminoma: dysplastic cells in adjacent tubule. This is an abnormal tubule filled with highly atypical cells. It is close to a seminoma. It may represent invasion of the seminoma along the tubule but there are claims that such lesions represent *in situ* malignant change which occurs before the development of invasive germ-cell tumours. *(H&E × 256)*

1308

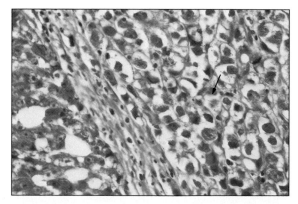

1308 Combined seminoma and teratoma. The right side of the field shows a tumour with the appearances of a seminoma (arrowed),while the left side shows a teratoma. Where such combinations occur, the tumour has the prognosis of the teratoma. *(H&E × 160)*

1309

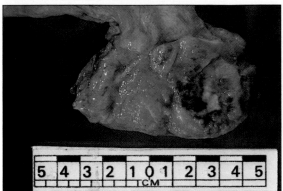

1309 Teratoma. Section through a testis containing a tumour showing widespread areas of haemorrhage and necrosis.

1310

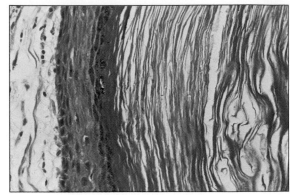

1310 Teratoma: differentiated (WHO equivalent: teratoma mature or immature). Part of a tumour showing differentiation along many cell lines all of them being well-differentiated tissue with no evidence of malignancy. This area shows a well-differentiated stratified squamous epithelium which is keratinising. Though all elements appear benign the behaviour of some of these tumours is malignant. *(H&E × 160)*

1311

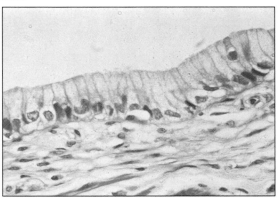

1311 Teratoma: differentiated (WHO equivalent: teratoma mature or immature). Another area of the tumour shown in **1310**, but this shows a well-differentiated mucus-secreting epithelium. In children this type of tumour may contain immature elements which do not imply malignancy. *(H&E × 160)*

1312

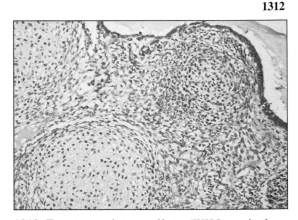

1312 Teratoma: intermediate (WHO equivalent: embryonal carcinoma and teratoma with malignant transformation). A malignant teratoma containing incompletely differentiated tissue and cells having the features of malignancy. This section shows cuboidal epithelium in the top right corner; there is poorly formed cartilage in the bottom left corner and incompletely differentiated tissue between. *(H&E × 64)*

1313

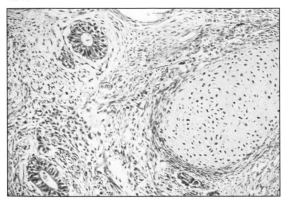

1313 Malignant teratoma: intermediate (WHO equivalent: embryonal carcinoma and teratoma or teratoma with malignant transformation). Similar to **1312** with cartilage, glands and undifferentiated tissue. *(H&E × 64)*

1314

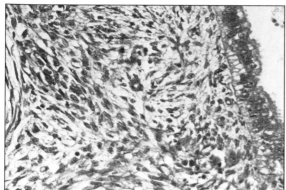

1315

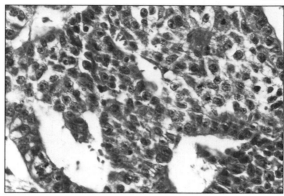

1314 Malignant teratoma: intermediate (WHO equivalent: embryonal carcinoma and teratoma or teratoma with malignant transformation). Higher magnification showing an epithelium with cellular atypicality and stroma with mitotic figures. *(H&E × 160)*

1315 Malignant teratoma: undifferentiated (WHO equivalent: embryonal carcinoma). A malignant teratoma lacking mature elements but which has a variable appearance, often with some differentiation suggesting an adenocarcinoma. *(H&E × 256)*

1316 Malignant teratoma trophoblastic. This testis shows a haemorrhagic mass at one pole. This was composed predominantly of trophoblastic tissue.

1316

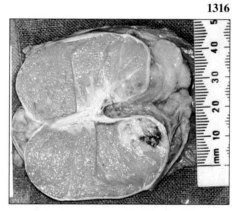

1317

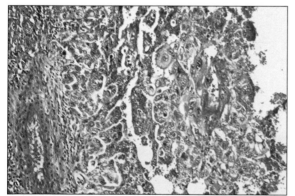

1318

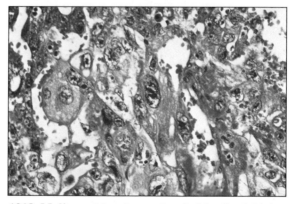

1317 Malignant teratoma: trophoblastic (WHO equivalent: choriocarcinoma alone or with embryonal carcinoma or other germ-cell tumour). A malignant teratoma with extra-embryonic differentiation to trophoblast. The section shows cyto- and syncytio-trophoblast arranged in a villous pattern. *(H&E × 64)*

1318 Malignant teratoma: trophoblastic. A higher magnification of the specimen in **1317** to show syncytiotrophoblast. Trophoblastic differentiation in a teratoma carries a worse prognosis. *(H&E × 256)*

1319

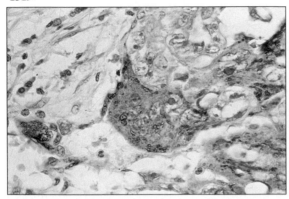

1319 Malignant teratoma: trophoblastic. This type of tumour was one of the first to be associated with a 'tumour marker' detectable in the serum or urine, human chorionic gonadotrophin (HCG). The hormone produced by the tumour cells may also be demonstrated in the tissue by the use of labelled antiserum to the tumour product. In this section HCG has been demonstrated by using antiserum to its ß subunit to localise an enzyme, a peroxidase, to the HCG-containing cells: the peroxidase produces a brown reaction product from a substrate. The brown stain represents sites where HCG is present. *(Immunoperoxidase immunocytochemistry for HCG × 256)*

1320

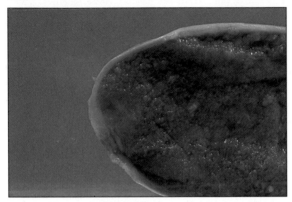

1320 Malignant teratoma. Occasionally a primary tumour may scar up while metastases kill the patient. This testis comes from a patient who died with widespread metastases arising from a malignant teratoma. The only lesion seen in either testis was this thin scar at one pole of the left testis.

1321

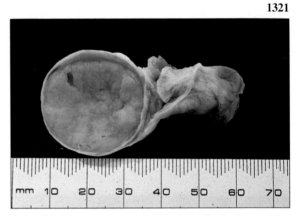

1321 Yolk-sac tumour (synonyms include: orchioblastoma, endodermal sinus tumour, adenocarcinoma of the infant testis). Pure yolk-sac tumours tend to occur in infants. This is one in a child of 9 months. The cut surface shows a well-circumscribed yellowish tumour. Yolk-sac elements may be found in adult teratomas and tend to be associated with a poorer prognosis: like trophoblastic elements, they represent extra-embryonic development of a teratoma.

1322

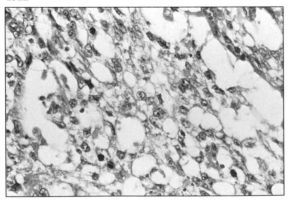

1322 Yolk-sac tumour. The tumour typically grows in a pattern of a loose vacuolated network with apparent glandular differentiation which gave rise to its designation as 'adenocarcinoma'. *(H&E × 160)*

1323

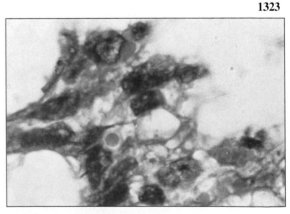

1323 Yolk-sac tumour. A higher magnification shows the eosinophilic globules in the cytoplasm of cells. The globules can be shown to contain AFP, an oncofoetal antigen which may also be present in the serum of patients with this tumour.

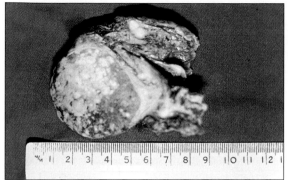

1324 Interstitial-cell tumour (Leydig-cell tumour). These tumours are yellow to brown on naked-eye examination; they measure up to 10cm in diameter and are often lobulated. They may be hormonally active, tending to give virilisation in childhood and feminisation in adults. Most are benign but about 10 per cent metastasise.

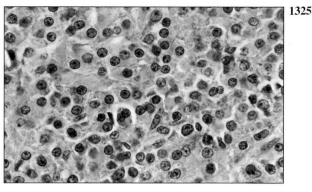

1325 Interstitial-cell tumour (Leydig-cell tumour). The tumour consists of regular polygonal cells with eosinophilic or vacuolated cytoplasm. The nuclei are round to oval and contain small nucleoli. Large cells which are sometimes binucleate or multinucleate are occasionally present. *(H&E × 256)*

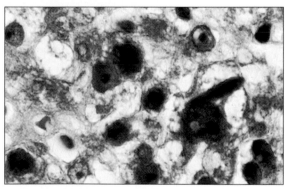

1326 Interstitial-cell tumour: Reinke crystalloids. These cytoplasmic inclusions are a marker of interstitial cells. They are rod-shaped structures that are difficult to see with haematoxylin and eosin, but more easily demonstrated with Masson's trichrome. They are seen in less than half of interstitial-cell tumours. *(Masson's trichrome × 640)*

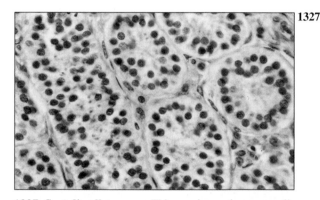

1327 Sertoli-cell tumour. This specimen shows a well-differentiated Sertoli-cell tumour with clear cells arranged in a tubular fashion; less well-differentiated tumours cause diagnostic problems. Their behaviour is usually benign but metastasis can occur. *(H&E × 256)*

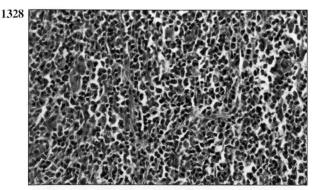

1328 Testis: malignant lymphoma. The testis may be the site of a primary malignant lymphoma or it may be secondarily involved in a generalised lymphoma. It tends to occur in older patients. This tumour shows sheets of small darkly staining cells with little cytoplasm. This is a lymphosarcoma. *(H&E × 160)*

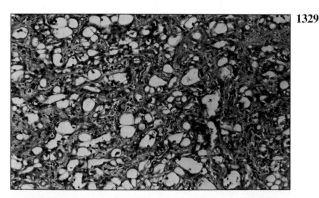

1329 Adenomatoid tumour. This is the commonest tumour of paratesticular tissues and is benign. They are small, usually asymptomatic nodules. This section shows that it is composed of gland-like structures and stroma. *(H&E × 160)*

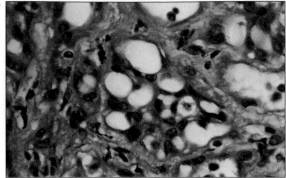

1330 Adenomatoid tumour. A higher magnification of the tumour in picture **1329** showing the characteristic mixture of connective tissue and spaces lined by flattened or cuboidal cells, some of which are vacuolated. The term 'mesothelioma' is sometimes loosely applied to these lesions. True mesothelioma may rarely occur in the tunica vaginalis and is a malignant tumour, more often seen in pleura and peritoneum. *(H&E × 256)*

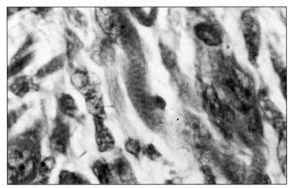

1331 Paratesticular rhabdomyosarcoma. Although it is rare, this tumour is relatively common among paratesticular malignancies. The histological pattern varies, but this section shows strap-like cells with pleomorphic nuclei and cross-striations in the cytoplasm of some cells. *(H&E × 640)*

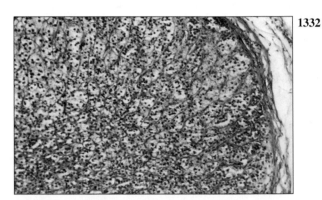

1332 Spermatic cord: adrenal rest. These developmental abnormalities may occur in the spermatic cord or in the rete testis. The arrangement of cells resembles that of the zona fasciculata in the adrenal cortex. They are quite benign. *(H&E × 64)*

Testicular tubule morphology

Illustration of the many lesions seen in the testes of the subfertile male is beyond the scope of this work, but some of the commoner lesions are illustrated below. In biopsy of the testis for an assessment of morphology, formol saline is an inadequate fixative because it causes considerable distortion and poor preservation. Bouin's fluid gives much better preservation.

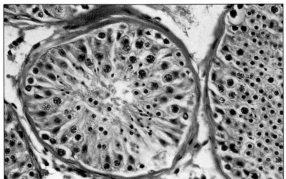

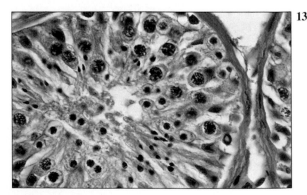

1333 and 1334 Testis: normal. Testicular tubules with Sertoli cells and germ cells with maturation through spermatocytes and spermatids to spermatozoa (in the centre of the tubule). The basement membrane and associated connective tissue is of normal size. The intertubular connective tissue is loose and interstitial cells are not prominent. (**1333** *(H&E × 160)*; (**1334** *H&E × 256)*)

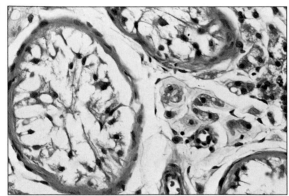

1335 Undescended testis. The tubules in this specimen are lined by Sertoli cells and no spermatogenesis is apparent. The tubular basement membranes are hyalinised and there is peritubular fibrosis. Interstitial cells are prominent. *(H&E × 160)*

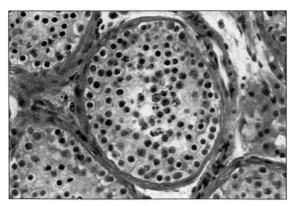

1336 Testis: maturation arrest. In this abnormality maturation of spermatozoa is halted and failure of spermatogenesis results. These tubules show Sertoli cells, germ cells and spermatocytes but virtually nothing beyond that. *(H&E × 160)*

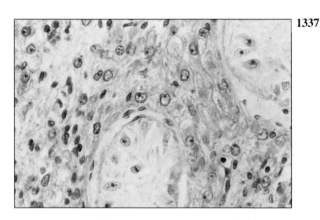

1337 Testis: Klinefelter's syndrome. This biopsy (from a chromatin-positive Klinefelter's syndrome) shows tubules lined with Sertoli cells, hyalinised basement membranes and no spermatogenesis. There are very prominent masses of interstitial cells. *(H&E × 160)*

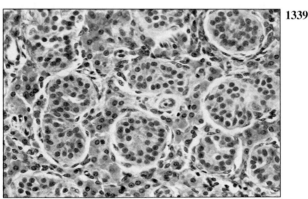

1338 Testis: post-mumps orchitis. This biopsy came from a subfertile patient with a history of mumps orchitis. There were patchy lesions in the testis where, as illustrated by this section, tubules showed atrophy of lining cells, marked hyalinisation of the basement membrane and fibrosis of the interstitial tissue. *(H&E × 160)*

1339 Testis: testicular feminisation. This term refers to the syndrome of a genetic male with a female body form and external genitalia but with no uterus or tubes and little axillary and pubic hair. The testis is composed of small tubules with no spermatogenesis; they are immature and similar to those in the prepubertal male. The interstitial cells are very prominent. *(H&E × 160)*

Further reading

Chapter 1
Magnetic resonance imaging
1. Hricak H, Crooks L, Sheldon P and Kaufman L, 1983. Nuclear Magnetic Resonance of the Kidney. *Radiology* **146**: 425–432.
2. Sommer F G, McNeal J E and Carrol C L, 1986. MR depiction of zonal anatomy of the prostate at 1.5T. *J Comput Assist Tomogr* **10**: 983–989.

Positron emission tomography
1. Strauss L G and Conti P S, 1991. The application of PET in Clinical Oncology. *J Nuc Med* **32**: 623–648.
2. Hawkins R A, Hoh C, Glaspy J, *et al.*, 1992. The Role of Positron Emission Tomography in Oncology and Other Whole Body Applications. *Seminars in Nuclear Medicine* **22**: 268–284. Philadelphia, USA: W B Saunders & Co.

Chapter 2
1. Mandell J, Blyth B, Peters C A, Retik A B, Estnoll J A and Benacerral B R, 1991.The Natural History of Structural Genito-urinary Defects Detected in utero. *Radiology* **178**: 193.
2. R H Whitaker, 1990. *Congenital Abnormalities of the Urinary Tract. An illustrated guide.* Edinburgh, London, Melbourne and New York: Churchill Livingstone.

Chapter 3
1. Mandel G L, Claisson R E and Volberding P A, 1990. Clinical Manifestations of HIV infection. In: Douglas R G J and Bennett J E (eds) *Principles and Practice of Infectious Diseases.* New York: Churchill Livingstone.
2. Leport C, Rousseau F, Perconne C, Salmon D, Joerg A and Vilde J, 1988. Bacterial Prostatitis in patients infected with the human immunodeficiency virus. *J Urol* **141**: 334–336.
3. Slevcluk M, de Silza M, Armenakas N, Tonnerbaum M and Fracchia J. 1989. The Male Genital Tract in AIDS (abstract 138) Eighty-fourth Annual Meeting of the American Urological Association. *J Urol* **141**: 354A.

Chapter 4
Gow J G, 1992. Genitourinary tuberculosis. In: Walsh P C, Retik A B, Stamey T A and Vaughan Jr E D (eds) *Campbell's Urology 6th edn.* Philadelphia, USA: W B Saunders & Co. pp 951–981.

Chapter 5
1. Smith J H, Lichtenberg Franz Von, Lehaman J S, 1992. Urinary Schistosomiasis. In: Walsh P C, Retik A B, Stamey T A and Vaughan Jr E D (eds) *Campbells Urology 6th edn.* Philadelphia, USA: W B Saunders Co. pp 883–906.
2. Cline B L, Richards F O, El alamy M A, El Haks, Ruiz-Tiber, Hughes J M and McNeeley D F, 1989. Nile Delta Schistosomiasis. Survey 48 years after Scott. *Am J Trop Med Hyg* **47:** 56.

Chapter 6
1. Chisholm G D and Fair W R (eds), 1990. *Scientific Foundations in Urology, Urolithiasis Section IV.* pp 170–223. Oxford: Heinemann Medical Books; Chicago: Year Book Medical Publishers Inc.
2. Resnick M I and Pak Charles Y C, 1990. *Urolithiasis: A Medical and Surgical Reference.*Philadelphia, USA: W B Saunders & Co.

Chapter 7
Renal Oncocytoma
Lieber M M, 1990. Renal oncocytoma prognosis and treatment. *Eur Urol* **18**(2): 17.
Endometriosis
Lucero S P, Wise H A, Kirsh G, Devoe K, Hess M C, Kandawalla N and Drago J R, 1988. Ureteric obstruction secondary to endometriosis. Report of 3 cases and review of the literature. *Br J Urol* **61:** 201.

Chapter 8
Industrial bladder cancer
Steinbeck G, Plato N, Nosell S E *et al.*, 1990. Urothelial cancer and some industrial related chemicals. An evaluation of the epidemiologic literature. *Am J Ind Med* **17**: 371.

Chapter 9
Diagnosis
Cooler W H, 1991. Prostatic Specific Antigen, Digital Rectal Examination and Transurethral Ultrasonic Examination of the Prostate in Prostatic Cancer. *Monogr Urol* **12**: 3.

Chapter 10
1. Turner-Warwick R T, 1989. Prevention of complication resulting from pelvic fracture urethral injuries and from their surgical management. *Urol Clin North Am* **16**: 335.
2. Devine C J, Jordan G H and Devine P C, 1989. Primary realignment of the disrupted prostatomembranous urethra. *Urol Clin North Am* **16**: 291.

Chapter 11
Varicocele
Peng B C H, Tomashelsky P and Nagler H M, 1990. The cofactor effect. *Varicocele & Infertility Fertil Steril.* **5A**: 143.
Neoplasms of the testis
Ritchie J P, 1992, Neoplasms of the Testis. In: Walsh P C, Retik A B, Stamey T A and Vaughan Jr E D (eds) *Campbell's Urology 6th edn.* Philadelphia, USA: W B Saunders & Co. pp 1222–1263.

Chapter 12
Impotence
Golstein I, and Krane R J, 1992. Diagnosis and therapy of erectile dysfunction. In: Walsh P C, Retik A B, Stamey T A and Vaughan Jr E D (eds) *Campbells Urology 6th Edition.* Philadelphia, USA: W B Saunders & Co. pp 3033–3070.

Index

Numbers in **bold** refer to figure numbers, numbers in *italics* refer to page numbers of tables, and all other numbers are page numbers.

C

KUB
calculus in horseshoe kidney, **575–578**
calculus in pelviureteric junction obstruction, **579–581**
calyceal calculus, **565–566, 571–572**
stasis stone in calyceal diverticulum, **567–568**
ureteric calculi, **618, 625**

L

Lasertripsy, 129
Leiomyosarcoma, **771–775**
histology, **775**
Lesch–Nyhan syndrome, *127*
Leukoplakia, **361–363**
Lipomatosis, pelvic, **317–319**
Lithotripsy, 129, 148
ballistic, 129
Lymphadenopathy
para-aortic, **1280–1283**
prostate carcinoma metastases, **1064**
Lymphangiography, testicular tumour, **1278–1279**
Lymphography, **40**
Lymphoma
kidney, **780**
malignant of testis, **1328**

M

MAG3 renogram, **60–63**
pelvic kidney, **157**
Magenta, 212, **954**
Magnetic resonance imaging (MRI), **45–47**
kidney cysts, **791**
oncocytoma, **750–751**
renal tumour, **724–726**
Wilm's tumour, **759–760**
Malakoplakia, 157, **373–383**
histology, **381–383**
Michaelis–Gutmann bodies, **382–383**
vesical plaques, **374–378**
Malignancy, *127*
Matrix stone, 128
Megaureter, 43, **229–230**
renal calculi, **582–583**
Metanephric blastema, 45
4,4'–Methylenebis (2–chloroaniline) (MBOCA), 212
Micturating cystourethrogram (MCU), vesicoureteric reflux, **260–264, 266–267, 271, 274**
Micturition
bladder during, **126**
Micturition
pressure–flow study, **127**
urethra during, **126**
Mucoprotein, 128
Mycobacterium tuberculosis, 96, 97

N

1–Naphthylamine, 212, 213, **953**
2–Naphthylamine, 212, **953**
Nephroblastoma, 157, 159, **755–770**
Nephrocalcinosis, **588, 589–592**
with stone street, **592**
Nephrogram, dense, **644, 712**
Nephrostogram, **50, 646**
Nephrostomy tube, **616**

O

Oligohydramnios, 43
Oncocytoma, 157, 169, **747–751**
cartwheel appearance, **749**
Osteoclasis, 132
Osteoporosis, 132, **555**
Oxalate crystals, **89–90**

P

Paget's disease
of bone, *127*, **1057, 1067**
of the penis, **1194–1195**
Pancreas
diffuse calcification, **562**
with staghorn calculus, **560**
Pancreatectomy, *127*
Papaverine Doppler ultrasound, **1173–1174**
penile, **59**
Papillary necrosis, **309–313**
calcification, **593–594**
Paraphimosis, **1180–1184**
Parathyroid, hyperplasia, 132
Pelvic lipomatosis, **317–319**
Pelvicalyceal system, **50**
blind calyx abnormality, **192–193**
Pelviureteric junction (PUJ)
calculi, **579–581**
intravenous urogram (IVU), **579–580**
congenital, **579–580**
obstruction, 43, **68, 194–216**
infection, **210, 215–216**
intravenous urogram, **195**
megaureter, **230**
renography in diagnosis, 57, **203–205**
rupture, **211**
Whitaker test, **206–209**
Penis
balanitis, **1144–1145**
balanitis xerotica obliterans, **1182–1193**
Buschke–Löwenstein lesion, **1158–1159**
chancre of syphilis, **1146**
corpora cavernosography, **1170–1172, 1176–1177**
dermoid cyst, **1160–1163**

Radionuclide
    cystography, 26
    DMSA scanning in vesicoureteric reflux, **275–277**, **279**
    MAG3, **60–63**
    renal scanning, 24, **60–66**
Red cells
    dysmorphic, **91**
    sickle–shaped, **92**
Renal agenesis, 43, 45, **143**
Renal arteriography, **34–38**
Renal artery stenosis, 188, **843–853**
    fibroelastic internal proliferation, **851**
    fibromuscular hyperplasia, **844**
    glomeruli in atrophic tubules, **852**
    juxtaglomerular apparatus hyperplasia, **835**
    nephrectomy specimen, **850**
    post-stenotic dilatation, **845**
    stricture, **845–846**
Renal biopsy, **49**
Renal cyst disease, **797**
    see also Kidney, cysts
Renal surgery, percutaneous, 129
Renal tubular acidosis, **588**
Renal tumours, 157, 158–159, **700**
    adenocarcinoma, 157
    calcification, **700**
    carcinoma, 157
    cortical carcinoma, 157, 167, **735–746**
        aspiration biopsy, **746**
        cell growth patterns, 167, **739–745**
        histology, **739–745**
    pelvic, 157, **700**
    see also Kidney, tumours
Renal ultrasound, **1–6**
Renogram, pelviureteric obstruction, **203–205**
Renography, renal artery stenosis, **848–849**
Retrograde pyelography, **31–32**
    hydronephrosis, **198**
    ureteric calculi, **619**
    ureteric duplication, **150**
Retroperitoneal fibrosis (RPF), idiopathic, 81, **324–336**
    ascending ureterography, **327–328**, **332–334**
    double pigtail stent, **331**
    histopathology, **335–336**
    intravenous urogram, **332–334**
    in para–aortic inflammatory disease, **330**
Rigid cystoscopy
bladder tumour, **877**
prostate, **1017**

S

Sarcoidosis, *127*
Scanning electron microscopy, **90**
Schistosomiasis *see* Bilharzia
Scrotum
    epithelial cysts, **1219–1220**
    oil cancers, **1221–1222**

Scrotum *cont.*
    spindle–cell sarcoma, **1223–1224**
    ultrasonography, 269
    wart, **1217–1218**
Seminal vesicles
    bilharzia, **539–540**
    transrectal ultrasound, **11**
    tuberculosis, **474**
Seminal vesiculogram, **41**
Sickle–cell disease, **92**
    papillary necrosis, **309–310**
Spermatic cord, adrenal rest, **1332**
Sphincter, external, **98**
    spastic, **129**, **131**
Splenic artery, ring shadow, **561**
Steine strasse *see* Stone street
Stents
    double pigtail in retroperitoneal fibrosis, **331**
    ureteric, **55**, **650–654**
Steroid therapy, *127*
Stone analysis, 128
Stone disease, management, 148
Stone formers, 127, *128*
    hyperparathyroidism, 132
Stone street, **592**, **617**
    extra shock wave lithotripsy, **616**
    ureteric, **654**
Stress incontinence, **133**

T

T-helper lymphocytes, 95
^{99m}Tc DMSA static scans, 25, **64–6**
Testis, **85–87**
    adrenal rest, **1332**
    appendage, **1230–1232**
    colour Doppler scan, **14**, **1265**
    CT scan of inpalpable, **1273–1274**
    ectopic, 257
    feminisation syndrome, **1339**
    granulomatous orchitis, **1258**
    histology, **1333–1339**
    hydrocele, 269, **1225–1229**, **1241**
    inflammation, **1248**
    inguinal, **1271**
    Klinefelter's syndrome, **1337**
    maldescent, **1269–1274**
        histology, **1272**
    maturation arrest, **1336**
    normal, **1333–1334**
    orchitis, post-mumps, **1338**
    spermatocele, **1238**
    torsion, **1250–1257**
        histology, **1257**
    tuberculous epididymitis, **486**
    tubule morphology, **1333–1339**